SCARY DIAGNOSIS

Navigating Fear, Finding Strength, and Securing the Health Care You Deserve

EDWARD G. ROGOFF

Prospecta Press

Copyright © 2025 by Edward G. Rogoff

ALL RIGHTS RESERVED. No part of this work covered by the copyright may be reproduced or used in any form or by any means—graphic, electronic, or mechanical, including photocopying, recording, taping, Web distribution or information storage and retrieval systems—without the written permission of Edward G. Rogoff.

Hardcover ISBN 978-1-63226-151-9
eBook ISBN 978-1-63226-152-6

PUBLISHED BY PROSPECTA PRESS
P.O. Box 3131
Westport, CT 06880

www.prospectapress.com

Book and cover design by Alexia Garaventa

Manufactured in the United States of America

To Perry-Lynn, the love of my life

Contents

Acknowledgments   *vii*

Introduction   1

Chapter 1: The First Shock, Then Waiting for Answers   **8**
When you receive a scary diagnosis, you need to know how to receive it, hear it, process it, and rely on others to provide prospective.

Chapter 2: Life or Death   **13**
Everyone eventually dies, and some diagnoses are death sentences. But for almost every diagnosis there is a reason for more optimism than pessimism.

Chapter 3: Vulnerability Squared   **18**
Being sick makes you feel vulnerable, fearful, and powerless.

Chapter 4: Sick Children   **34**
As vulnerable as you are as an adult, children are far more defenseless.

Chapter 5: Building Your Team   **50**
When you receive a scary diagnoses, you naturally tend to become depressed and isolate yourself from the world.

Chapter 6: You Must Never Lose Your Dignity   **57**
At its worst, medical treatment can feel like torture, creating unimaginable pain that can reduce you to feeling like a supplicant begging for relief.

Chapter 7: Distrust and Suspicion   65
Skepticism is good; paranoia is bad. But you are likely somewhere on this continuum.

Chapter 8: Selecting and Managing Your Doctor   72
How you can find and select the right doctor.

Chapter 9: Faith, Hope, and the Three Stooges   84
You need to focus on your attitude and take concrete steps to keep your mood positive.

Chapter 10: To Share or Not to Share   92
It may be painful to share, but it can also bring you relief.

Chapter 11: Managing the Hospital Experience   97
Which hospital you should select to receive the best care?

Chapter 12: Coping with Big, Bad Bureaucracies   106
How the bureaucracies of insurance companies, hospitals, medical practices, and government programs can crush your spirit and damage your chances of successful treatment.

Chapter 13: Confront Your Disease by Being More Than Just a Patient   123
Being engaged in your work, family, and interests is what makes you who you are and you shouldn't lose that to your scary diagnosis.

Chapter 14: With Gratitude, Optimism Is Sustainable   136
You must strive to find gratitude and acknowledge the strength you found when coping with your scary diagnosis.

Suggested Reading   *145*

Index   *147*

Acknowledgments

While there may be one author's name on the cover of *Scary Diagnosis*, the reality is that many people played essential roles in this book's creation: my family and friends who have provided care and support throughout my life as I dealt with hemophilia, liver disease, and the liver transplant form the essential team to manage these various and difficult issues. These include my wife, Perry-Lynn, and our children, David and Justine.

Dr. Christopher Walsh was my hematologist for many years and offered expert and supportive care as I dealt with hemophilia and then liver disease. He is the rare physician who is both an empathetic caregiver and an accomplished scientist. When my liver disease progressed, Dr. Walsh introduced me to the hepatologist Dr. Leona Kim-Schluger, whose brilliance and dedication provides a model for any physician. Dr. Kim-Schluger, in turn, introduced me to Dr. Charles Miller, who runs the transplant program at the Cleveland Clinic, where I received the highest level of care I could imagine. Dr. Federico Aucejo of the Cleveland Clinic's surgical team lead the surgery itself.

This book wouldn't have made it to the first chapter without the support and guidance of Dr. Andrew Aronson. After more than fifty years of silence on the painful issues of my hemophilia and its difficult treatment I experienced as a child, Dr. Aronson supported me in opening up to them and coming to terms with this painful past. This book is the natural outgrowth of my meetings with him.

During the last two years, I lost two wonderful and supportive friends: Alvin Puryear and Rich Rosenstein. They provided guidance and wise counsel as this book progressed from an idea to a manuscript. I miss them every day.

Mike Shatzkin, my friend for decades, is a publishing consultant who understands every aspect of this complex and rapidly changing industry. Without Mike's help, there would be no book. Mike introduced me to his publisher, David Wilk of Prospecta Press, who has been a wise and active partner in creating *Scary Diagnosis*.

Among the ways Mike provided great help was by introducing me to George Gibson, the brilliant executive editor of Grove Atlantic. George had recently published Dr. Mike Magee's *Code Blue: Inside America's Medical Industrial Complex*, the wonderful overview of the health-care system. George immediately saw the need and proper positioning for *Scary Diagnosis* and gave me meaningful encouragement that was essential in the book's development.

As the book took shape, I shared drafts with readers who could give me wise and no-holds-barred feedback. Dr. Elyse Morgan, a friend of more than fifty years, is a brilliant psychologist whose feedback was crucial in the book's evolution. Dana Isaacson provided feedback on early drafts and helped me define the purpose and audience for the book.

Other readers have included Bob Wolf, a leading expert on a wide range of issues related to seniors; David Roth and Rick

Bacher, the most capable marketing and design executives I know; my academic colleague Stuart Schulman; my dear friend Ilene Masser, a therapist who has experienced more than her share of scary diagnoses among her family and her patients; and Barbara Knothe, who started her career as an intensive care nurse and then became an incredibly knowledgeable attorney specializing in health and medical issues. Karen Shatzkin, a brilliant intellectual property attorney, provided clear and valuable information to manage those issues. My friend and former student, Elisa Balabram, has developed into a wonderful writer and I am grateful for her thoughtful feedback.

Valuable feedback came from my cousins Marty Greenfield and Miriam Karash, and from Thom Harrington, with whom I worked for thirty years in his capacity as the executive director of the Hemophilia Association of New York.

Throughout this project and every other project, I have worked on over the last forty years, my partner has been my wife, Perry-Lynn Moffitt. When I met her and fell in love, I appreciated her beauty, caring personality, and commitment to family. Only later did I realize that she is a brilliant and talented writer and editor. She started with reading and editing my doctoral dissertation in 1980 and her pencil has made countless improvements. I could not have brought these projects to fruition without her.

As you progress through *Scary Diagnosis* you will meet eight people and their families who have dealt with difficult health issues and have provided candid and insightful experiences. These include Michael Hamilton, Don and Jeanne Schepers, Deborah Dokken, Mark Gibbel, Ethan Skinner, Adam Greathouse, and Ava Barron and her parents. I am filled with gratitude for their contributions.

INTRODUCTION

"This is a very serious condition."

"You now need to make this the number one focus of your life."

"Don't jump to the conclusion that this is a death sentence."

A meeting with your doctor that includes startling language such as the above statements marks the beginning of a daunting journey. You must come to terms with crushing fear while transitioning from a regular person to a patient. And while you cope with the various weapons medical science aims at your physical condition, you must also deal with some of the largest bureaucracies in the world—insurance companies, hospitals, Medicare, Medicaid—*and* simultaneously manage helpful or nonhelpful family and friends.

The purpose of this book is to help you as you or a loved one face long, complex, and often difficult medical conditions and treatments. From grand hospital atriums that rival Las Vegas casinos to the smallest pill that challenges your eyesight and dexterity to maneuver into your mouth, the health-care system seems to remind us again and again that we are inadequate and definitely not in charge.

But *you* are in charge, and don't you forget it.

More often than not, patients cannot adequately manage this overly complex process or take in all the information they receive from the legion of medical professionals they encounter. Sometimes a patient relies disproportionately on one doctor's advice. It's no surprise that under such emotionally fraught circumstances, someone might make a bad decision or avoid making important decisions altogether.

To avoid being overwhelmed by the medical system, patients must maintain their autonomy while gaining a modicum of control over their treatments. The last thing any sick person needs is to feel further victimized or even more anxious.

I have a lifetime of experience managing my chronic illness and long-term treatments. Along the way I have made my share of mistakes, but I have also learned valuable lessons. I want to use this knowledge to help others. But this book is not about me. Instead, my vast experience in the health-care system merely provides examples of the various issues that you may face. I offer coping strategies when dealing with diseases and their treatments.

On July 23, 2011, I woke up in Cleveland, Ohio, to find myself cured of hemophilia, liver cancer, and cirrhosis. During the following year, I would also be cured of hepatitis C. But my life as a patient began long before that, when I was two years old and first diagnosed with hemophilia, the bleeder's disease.

As a patient, you may be confronted with major decisions in areas in which you are ill prepared. It's not unusual to delegate these decisions to professionals, people who may or may not have your best interests at heart and who—let's be honest—sometimes make mistakes.

My parents were from a generation that deified doctors. They accepted the opinions of medical professionals without challenge and followed their instructions in every detail. They waited without complaint for hours if the doctor was late, they never sought a second opinion, and they rarely asked challenging questions.

I would grow up to develop a totally different attitude. I remember the first time I felt that a doctor had no idea what he was talking about. I was six years old and we were at our summer house in New Jersey. I was using a tricycle as a scooter, with one foot on the back and one pushing along the ground. I slipped, and my left leg slid off the back and bashed into the trike as I tried to stop it. Within minutes I had a huge bump on my shin. Within hours I had a large blue-and-purple bruise that covered half of my shin. It felt warm, and it hurt.

A doctor lived a few doors down, and my mother asked him to stop over and take a look. He arrived in red shorts and carrying his leather doctor's bag, which I imagined was filled with needles. My mother pulled back the sheet covering my colorful leg. As a hemophiliac, I'd seen many bruises and they didn't scare me, but the doctor gasped.

"Maybe this one was really different," I thought.

"How long has he had hemophilia?" he asked.

Even as a six-year-old, I knew that hemophilia is mostly a genetic disease that manifests shortly after birth or at a very young age. "This dope knows nothing," I thought for the first time in my life.

I pulled my leg back under the sheet.

But the doctor, like many others, didn't feel his job was done unless he dispensed a drug. He reached into his bag and took out a glass container with small white pills. He gave them to my mother and for the first time I heard the word *phenobarbital*.

I was given one of the pills and soon fell asleep. You might assume that phenobarbital is pain medication, but it's actually a sedative. The goal of this doctor's helpfulness was not to reduce my pain but to make me inactive and shut me up. Some doctors believe that taking some action—even the wrong action—is better than doing nothing.

I know I'm not perfect, but I suppose the fact that—against the odds—I am still alive, is evidence that I've done more right than wrong. But I've made mistakes, some major. I promise to be candid, and I will share my errors.

Once you enter the medical system, fear, denial, self-pity, and anger interfere with your ability to think clearly. It's hardly surprising that any one of us may be overwhelmed by emotions when faced with major decisions.

Also, you may be given conflicting advice from different sources. And you can bet that family and friends will have strong opinions, which you have to manage while remembering that your health-care decisions are your own.

Today's modern medical treatments may be ridiculed tomorrow. Once upon a time, applying leeches was cutting-edge medical treatment. (They're making a comeback, by the way.) Medical knowledge and what is regarded as "best practices" are constantly changing. Modern medicine can cure hundreds of diseases, reduce symptoms for diseases that can't be cured, and offer guidance and drugs to prevent serious problems. So, making these crucial and complex decisions in a world of rapidly evolving medical treatments and guidance is like playing Whac-a-Mole—with you as the mole.

Your goal is to identify the benefits that the medical system has to offer and to do so without too much wear and tear on your body.

Every person and institution you interact with has their own interests—many of them financial. Without understanding those interests, you cannot adequately manage your care. One of the purposes of this book is to explain how the individuals and institutions you are dealing with function while you're worrying about your health. Limiting liability, controlling costs, reducing overtime, pleasing drug companies, testing new treatments, and getting home in time for dinner are all issues that may be on your practitioner's mind while you are worried that you won't see your next birthday.

An example of self-interest at work: Insurance companies get paid a fixed amount upfront, and they work to pay out as little as possible. These mostly for-profit corporations are also competing with other insurance companies and operating in a highly regulated environment that includes Medicare, Medicaid, the Affordable Care Act (Obamacare), and many state programs. This competition among insurers is largely about what they charge in premiums, but it impacts the kinds of care they will pay for, which doctors and hospitals they will pay for—and ultimately how much of fees are the patient's responsibility.

Like many professionals, doctors are evaluated by patient satisfaction surveys, the number of days their patients stayed in the hospital after surgery, or the average number of minutes they spent with patients during visits. These outcome data are compared to those of other doctors in similar specialties or other programs with a similar focus. This leads to rankings that you may have seen advertised by some hospitals. These metrics are familiar to other professionals, but not to us.

For example, replacing a joint in a patient with a heart problem often means keeping the patient in the hospital longer to make sure their heart is fine. But that delay could increase a hospital's "average days in hospital post-surgery" statistic—a number the hospital wants to keep as low as possible. This may result in some doctors and hospitals being reluctant to take cases that will skew their statistical performance.

Another major metric for hospital performance is survival rates. Of course, it makes sense to track this statistic, but if a hospital tries to keep its survival rates high by rejecting sicker patients, seriously ill people will have trouble finding good care. In other words, the decisions of health-care organizations and professionals are based upon their own interests. This should be shocking but it's not. Your needs are often not at the top of their list.

After having been through more than my share of interactions with the health-care system, I became an advocate for patients.

I served—and still serve—on the board of the Hemophilia Association of New York; and I was its president for twenty-two years, including during the period when people with hemophilia were the group most seriously affected by HIV/AIDS—even more than gay men or intravenous drug users. I was a founder and president of an organization that beat the drug companies at their own game by obtaining discount drugs for patients with hemophilia; this organization now has more than $100 million in yearly revenue. I am also an advisor and board member of

Punkin' Futz, an organization that creates innovative products for children with learning disabilities. Between 2017 and 2024, I was a board member of LiveOnNY, which manages the organ transplant system in the New York City area and arranges around one thousand transplants annually.

Understanding the system will help you make better decisions, leading to improved health care and a better future. It is likely that you have chosen a doctor or hospital because of their reputation for knowledge and experience in the area that concerns you. Indeed, knowledge is power, but it works both ways. The more knowledge you have about the medical system, the doctors or hospitals you are considering for your care, and the disease or condition itself, the better you can manage your care.

Chapter 1

THE FIRST SHOCK, THEN WAITING FOR ANSWERS

I'm no mind reader, but I'm pretty certain you are reading this book because you are either waiting for test results or are trying to figure out what a recently received diagnosis means for your health, the health of a family member or friend, and your ability to live the life you want.

You may have never been in a place of such uncertainty before, but I hope this book can help you cope. After absorbing the shock of hearing a scary diagnosis, the time comes to map out a plan to manage it.

Some diagnoses are perfectly clear and virtually immediate. If you are in a car accident, have a heart attack, suffer a stroke, or have a painful kidney stone, a diagnosis will usually be made and confirmed within an hour, perhaps less. You can deal with treatments and will learn how your life will change. But some diagnoses never become clear. This is the case for one of the people you will meet as you read on, Adam Greathouse, a veteran who was gravely injured while serving on the NATO peacekeeping mission in Kosovo. Despite never receiving a definitive diagnosis, the story of his long struggle is both informative and inspiring.

Adam's condition was likely caused by some type of chemical poisoning. Some diagnoses are never clear. Autoimmune diseases such as lupus, rheumatoid arthritis, or psoriatic arthritis may forever surround you with swirling clouds of hypotheses proposed by doctors, your family, and the self-proclaimed experts on YouTube.

Conditions such as depression or migraine headaches will always be uncertain in origin and unpredictable as to when they flare up. Some questions that may never be answered could include:

- What caused this disease or symptoms?
- Are there any treatments that will cure it?
- Are there any treatments that will make me feel better?
- Does this disease progress and make me sicker?
- Will this become a chronic condition I need to live with for the rest of my life?

Even if these questions are answered, you will have to deal with a significant period of uncertainty until a clear diagnosis is made. For me, it was about six weeks from the MRI that brought the word *transplant* into my daily thoughts to the time I was placed on the transplant list waiting for a match that would cure my liver disease.

Adam, the veteran, was brought to the brink of death even though he never received a definitive diagnosis. Other patients discussed throughout this book visited multiple doctors in multiple specialties only to have some of the scariest diagnoses eliminated, but others that still held multiple dangers were left under active consideration.

Don, who you will meet in greater detail later in the book, is the son and grandson of men who developed Parkinson's disease late in life, so he was primed for indicators. When he noticed a tremor in his right hand as it hung by his side, he strongly suspected that it was Parkinson's, but it took a year and several doctors' appointments until he received a confirming diagnosis.

So here you stand looking past the teeth, down the throat, and into the belly of the beast. Jonah would spend three days and three nights in the belly of the whale that God had sent to save him from drowning. Then God had the whale burp up Jonah onto the beach. You should be so lucky. Jonah's journey took only three days, but that was because God didn't need prior authorization from an insurance company.

Perhaps you are motivated to go to the doctor because of pain or a skin spot that didn't look right. Your journey through the belly of the health-system beast may never have a clear ending. Do your best to come to terms with the process that will now control your thoughts and calendar.

1. You receive the doctor's first impression and hypotheses.

2. You await test results.

3. You see a specialist.

4. You await more test results.

5. You get a second opinion.

6. You await more test results.

7. You decide what action, if any, to take.

Brace yourself. Remember: you are strong. As dreadful as this sounds, prepare yourself for more of the same. One of the reasons you may get caught in a cycle of new doctors, new tests, and new conclusions is that medical diagnostic errors are shockingly common.

You might even say that this American tradition of diagnostic errors and mistreatments started with George Washington in 1799. At that time, the former president saw a doctor because he was feeling ill with a sore throat and chest congestion. Over the next few days, he was treated by four doctors who, with the patient's acquiescence, drained five pints of his blood—half the blood in the human body! To this day it's unclear if the extreme bloodletting killed Washington or if an undiagnosed infection proved fatal. Certainly removing half his blood was a major medical error and didn't help any possible recovery.

While bloodletting is no longer practiced, medical errors continue.

According to a 2014 report by the Society to Improve Diagnosis in Medicine (SIDM), an estimated 12 million people are affected by medical diagnostic errors in the US every year, resulting in the deaths of between 40,000 and 80,000 patients. Researchers estimate that about half of those errors could be "potentially harmful."

In a 2017 study of patients seeking second opinions from Mayo Clinic, researchers found that only 12 percent were correctly diagnosed by their primary care providers. More than 20 percent had been misdiagnosed, while 66 percent required some changes to their initial diagnoses.

A 2023 study by the National Institutes of Health estimated that diagnostic errors contribute to about 10 percent of patient deaths and "6 to 17 percent of adverse events in hospitals."

Some think that second opinions should be mandatory, but not all patients require second opinions. They raise the cost of care and slow down the process of beginning treatment. Some health insurers—in order to hold down costs—won't cover second opinions from experts outside their networks.

Reducing diagnostic errors means tackling human mistakes to traditional but flawed procedures for treating and diagnosing conditions.

How to Manage the First Steps

- Accept that you are beginning a process that will be long, complex, and frustrating.

- Be aware that mistakes are made and second opinions and visits to specialists can be worthwhile.

- Understand that you are now on a mission to get answers and you are in charge.

Chapter 2

LIFE OR DEATH

Receiving a scary diagnosis triggers fear. When I was told that I needed a liver transplant, my thoughts went to my death: What if I don't receive a new liver in time? What if I die in the process of receiving the transplant? What if I am not even accepted on the transplant list?

At the time, I was not thinking that a liver transplant would cure me and begin the healthiest period of my life—which was the case. As I waited for the process of becoming a transplant recipient to move ahead, going through my everyday life of teaching, working at the university, and seeing friends and family became an exercise of very pessimistic what-ifs.

"What if this is the last course I will teach? What if these are family members I will never see again?" Just walking through Central Park to go to a doctor's appointment triggered a "What if I never see Central Park in the spring again?"

After a few months, my thinking shifted to a more optimistic narrative. I was on the transplant list at Mount Sinai Hospital in New York, and although it might take a year to actually receive a liver, the doctors were optimistic that they could keep me alive that long. As a backup plan, they suggested I pursue getting on transplant lists at hospitals in other states that may have shorter waiting times. Their suggestions included the Cleveland Clinic, the University of Michigan Hospital, and Mayo Clinic. My home hospital of Mount Sinai is a world-class institution distinguished by great medical research and excellent patient care, but moving from one doctor's office to another is like walking through a maze. Over decades, Mount Sinai has grown in and around apartment houses, parking lots, and neighborhood schools.

When my wife and I traveled to the Cleveland Clinic to begin its intake process, my mood improved further. From my first day going through tests at the Cleveland Clinic, I thought I had been time-transported to the twenty-third century. The buildings had large spaces with clear directions and many red-jacketed guides to help. The waiting time for elevators was measured in seconds, robots delivered the mail, and valet parking helped those with limited mobility. The Cleveland Clinic prided itself on being the master of hospital logistics, calling its system "the Cleveland Clinic Way."

In one day, they took me through a battery of screening tests that had taken a week at Mount Sinai. When my CT scan ran four minutes late, the technician came out to apologize and explain that the previous patient had needed a few extra minutes. All this happy efficiency gave me confidence—and optimism. I began to feel that this was going to work out just fine. Bravo for great logistics.

Like me, Adam Greathouse benefited from being treated in one of the largest and most sophisticated logistical systems—in his case, the US military. Adam was injured, near death, and yet baffled his doctors. He had been moved from a Balkan battlefield to hospitals in Kosovo, then Germany, and at last to Walter Reed National Military Medical Center in Bethesda, Maryland. With each move, Adam accessed higher levels of care. There is little doubt that without fast decisions and the system in place to aid injured soldiers as quickly as possible, Adam would have died in Kosovo.

According to the American Society of Clinical Oncology, in 2022, 69 percent of people diagnosed with cancer lived five or more years since their diagnosis; 47 percent lived ten or more years since their diagnosis; and 18 percent lived twenty or more years since their diagnosis. Given that the life expectancy for the average sixty-five-year-old in the United States is 14.9 years, if you are diagnosed with cancer at that age, the disease's impact on your life expectancy may not be that great. Of course, nobody wants to go through the diagnosis process, the treatments, and being sick, but be aware that many cancer diagnoses are not death sentences.

Some of the greatest successes in cancer treatment have emerged from the treatment of childhood leukemia. Survival rates for most childhood cancers have improved—notably acute lymphoblastic leukemia, the most common childhood cancer. According to the American Cancer Society's *Cancer Facts & Figures 2023*, the five-year survival rate for acute lymphoblastic leukemia has increased from less than 10 percent in the 1960s to over 90 percent today due to improved treatment.

Heart problems such as cardiovascular disease, heart failure, and arrhythmias represent a broad array of diseases of different levels of severity. According to the Centers for Disease Control, in 2021, heart disease was the number one cause of death in the US, killing over 695,000 people. But many types of heart disease are subject to successful treatments. Cardiovascular disease, such as blocked arteries, can be treated by diet and exercise, insertions of stents to open the arteries, and bypass surgery in which the clogged arteries are replaced with clear arteries taken from other parts of the patient's body.

Patients with heart disease need to identify the specific disorders and the medical options. Overall, the life expectancy for patients who are diagnosed with heart disease is about seven years. But this varies greatly based on the type of disease and the treatments.

A large body of research has firmly established the significant influence that a positive mental attitude has on health outcomes. Specifically, among people with positive attitudes, immune systems are stronger, pain management more successful, surgical recovery times shorter, and the risk of developing cardiovascular disease reduced.

Achieving and maintaining a positive mental attitude is largely in your control.

Engaging in physical activity, interacting with people who are important to you, and laughing are all proven to improve your health and treatment outcomes.

Take Action Early

- Don't delay. Find a doctor and clinic that treats exactly what you have.
- Don't delay. Research strongly supports that earlier treatment is far more effective.
- Don't delay. If a doctor or clinic seems slow at making appointments or starting treatment, find a different doctor, clinic, or hospital.

- Focus on creating and supporting a good mood and positive outlook, even in the face of clearly negative outcomes.
- Take a look at the research and see if you have strong reasons for optimism.

Chapter 3

VULNERABILITY SQUARED

Steve Jobs changed the world. He and his partner Steve Wozniak basically invented the personal computer. From there, Jobs created the modern smartphone, tablet computers, and iTunes, and in his capacity as an investor and leader of Pixar, he advanced video animation to its present state. No one since Thomas Edison has more radically changed the world through technological advances.

In 2003, Jobs was diagnosed with a generally treatable form of pancreatic cancer. He delayed the normative treatments of drugs and surgery and instead used alternative medical approaches, including acupuncture, herbal remedies, and a vegan diet. These did not slow the progression of his cancer, and in 2004 he underwent pancreatic surgery.

But the cancer had already spread to his liver. In 2009, Jobs received a liver transplant. Two and a half years later, he died. Whether the pancreatic cancer had spread throughout his body or metastasized to his new liver has not been made public.

One of the richest people in the world with access to the best medical care, Jobs declined typical (and usually successful) treatments and in essence committed a slow suicide. I never met Jobs, but I have met other people who felt the attraction to alternative medical treatments.

Why would the brilliant, iconic, intellectual giant Steve Jobs, when confronted with a scary diagnosis, choose drinking organic beet juice over standard and proven medical treatments?

By many accounts, he was a difficult person. He was headstrong and intolerant of others. He was also extremely confident in his own judgment. You can see why a person such as Jobs would be reluctant to cede any control if the medical system made him feel vulnerable and powerless. Unlike most of us, this guy wasn't about to let any doctor or nurse demean him or—heaven forbid!—actually ignore his opinions. Instead, by following the alternative medicine regimen, Jobs believed that he could become his own doctor. He could choose less invasive treatments. He never had to leave his house.

This course of action worked just fine for his psyche but not for his body.

I don't want to sound negative about alternative medicine. I have availed myself of acupuncture for knee and hip pain and believe that it worked. I don't know if juicing cures anything, but it probably doesn't hurt.

But before you write off traditional medicine, let's recognize how much good it has done and—in all likelihood—can do for you. In the twentieth century, modern medicine has extended the average life span by thirty years. A person born in 1900 could expect to live to be forty-seven. Today, life expectancy is over seventy-seven. Bacterial infections such as pneumonia are now almost entirely curable, which allows for the miracle of organ transplants. Sure, I would rather drink a glass of carrot juice daily than submit to terrible chemotherapy, but chemotherapy can and does actually work.

Perhaps Jobs let himself be guided by his depression over being sick and rejected mainstream treatments. This encouraged decisions that, in hindsight, cost him his life. Jobs's biographer, Walter Isaacson, (*Steve Jobs,* Walter Isaacson, Simon and Schuster, 2011) who interviewed Jobs close to the end of his life, states that Jobs became aware that he'd made a fatal mistake.

I hope this book will help you make better decisions about your health.

Yes, life is fragile. We don't realize it until something unexpectedly reminds us. It may be the sudden loss of a friend or relative or our own scary diagnosis. Just how fragile we are was vividly exemplified by people in the streets wearing masks to protect themselves and others during the deadly worldwide COVID-19 pandemic.

Being sick, or being fearful of becoming sick, elicits all kinds of reactions, as it did with Jobs. Depression and denial top the list. Both magnify a patient's vulnerability, possibly rendering them immobilized by depression over being ill. Denial is often an immediate, short-term reaction to news that one can't cope with. The brain pushes the problematic news (or "reality" or "information") to the side, providing temporary relief from anxiety. But over time, denial will give the brain over to depression. Reality is creeping in and it must be recognized and dealt with, lest depression become much worse.

Choosing denial over action results in poor decision-making.

If we're in denial, we can maintain that everything's just hunky-dory and there's no reason to see a doctor. Avoidance is a typical and powerful emotional response to a scary diagnosis.

Inactivity can accompany depression, so even making an appointment to see a doctor is delayed. We come to illogical conclusions such as "I exercise and take vitamins, so I have nothing to worry about" or "My grandmother lived to 103, and she never took a pill."

Receiving a scary diagnosis triggers the stomach-churning anticipation of becoming sicker. We fear losing the ability to engage in activities we associate with joyful living, and, of course, we are afraid of dying. Depression can be a semi-catatonic, debilitating state for many. In its severe form, it can lead to thoughts of suicide and actual suicide.

Stay in bed, eat your favorite foods (if you eat anything), stream film noirs, and convince yourself that you will deal with it later. Been there. Done that. It doesn't work.

Don't waste time on denial. A mind-numbing rejection of reality is a perfect setup for depression to take hold. Instead, face facts, for better or worse, and make a plan.

Six Essential Strategies Following a Scary Diagnosis

1. **Start to build your team.** You cannot manage what's ahead all by yourself. You need support, experience, expertise, and love. Begin to consider who will be on your team.

2. **Start to build your tool kit.** Specific actions can help you prepare for the physical and psychological stresses that may lie ahead. For example, physical activity has proven to be more effective than antidepressants at improving one's mood. While you may not feel up to it during your upcoming treatment and recovery, exercise your body when you can. Psychological support from a therapist will be beneficial. Practicing meditation or engaging in other

activities you love, such as painting or baking, may be helpful. Be purposeful, but also give yourself a break now and then. Schedule time to occupy yourself with activities that will free your mind of scary thoughts.

3. **Research medical treatment options.** There are almost always options. Some doctors may urge aggressive treatment, beginning immediately, while others will counsel "watchful waiting." Which course of treatment you take is your decision. Take the time to create a strategy that includes a list of treatment options, treatment centers, and doctors.

4. **Join a Support Group.** Many hospitals, clinics, and patient associations run support groups for patients to learn from each other and share their experiences. Learning from the experiences of others and coming to understand that you are not alone, is tremendously helpful.

5. **Consider who will be in your inner circle.** Who will you tell what about your medical condition? From the time I was a child, my default decision has been to tell no one. There were reasons for this choice, but it is not an approach I recommend. On the other hand, some people who receive a scary diagnosis decide to wear a virtual sandwich sign announcing their condition to every family member, their colleagues at work, and anyone they sit next to on the bus. This also strikes me as extreme. In chapter 11 we'll discuss finding the right balance for you.

6. **Take the long view.** Remind yourself that someday you will look back on your life and appreciate that you found an inner strength you may not have known you had, which gave you the means to successfully cope with your condition and manage your care.

I thought of suicide once, when I was about fifty. I was being treated for hepatitis C with interferon, a drug that includes suicidal thoughts among its significant side effects.

When the first treatments for hepatitis C became available in the 1980s, interferon emerged as a leading drug of choice. Interferon is a naturally occurring protein made by the body that triggers a response to viral infections. Interferon starts the process that creates other proteins that interfere with the replication of the infecting virus—hence the name, interferon. It seemed logical to researchers that by loading up patients with interferon, the body would rally to destroy any viral invaders. With hepatitis C, it actually worked in about 10 percent of cases.

But for many people like me, the side effects were horrific. Interferon is administered by a shot under the skin. As someone with years of experience self-infusing clotting factor directly into my veins, I expected the interferon injection would be easy. But the twenty-four hours that followed each shot were not. The interferon triggered an intense flu-like reaction with aches, pains, fever, and chills. It made my skin dry and itchy, well beyond the help of cortisone creams. My red blood cell counts plummeted, which is akin to anemia, and produced extreme weakness.

Bad enough. But the worst side effect was depression. That caught me by surprise. No doctor had warned me to expect or even be prepared for it.

Later, as interferon treatment evolved, the drug was not administered until the patient had already begun a regimen of antidepressant drugs such as Prozac or Zoloft. But my experience took place before this had become standard operating procedure.

One day, as I was sitting—or should I say, slumping—in a chair in my living room, I participated in a rational-seeming discussion with myself about how I could commit suicide. I didn't own a gun, which in hindsight was a very good thing. I wasn't handy, so I couldn't imagine how to rig up a noose. Pills seemed easy, but I'd have to research which pills and find a doctor to prescribe them.

Then it hit me: Holy crap! I was actually thinking of suicide in a serious way.

I rallied my rationality and called a nurse practitioner at the hemophilia clinic whom I had known for many years. I told her suicide had just come into my mind, and it was no joke. She told me to stop the interferon and that we would discuss antidepressants if I later wanted to try interferon again. Certainly I was depressed about feeling lousy and frightened at my prospects, but these suicidal thoughts were a specific side effect of interferon. The experience gave me insight into how people can decide to end their lives in an unemotional way.

Whatever the cause, if you are depressed or suicidal, reach out for help. A friend, a relative may be there for you, or a medical professional could be even more useful.

Suffering in silence is boring and useless. Rally your forces and text a friend.

As we ingest increasing amounts of chemical medications, many of which have intense side effects and some of which interact with others, we must maintain an awareness of their potential impact on our complex bodily systems. We are, after all, a big vat of sloshing chemicals. You get crabby when you don't eat. And just maybe some of the drugs you take are adversely influencing your thoughts in a morbid way. If you are depressed, give this possibility serious thought.

Do not hesitate to ask your doctor or pharmacist about drugs' side effects or their possible interactions. Answers to these important questions can explain how you are feeling and impact your recovery.

Denial can push fear, anxiety, or depression away. The mind's ability to suppress thoughts, push unwanted emotions away, and carry on as if nothing were happening is astonishing. Denial can take feelings of vulnerability and push them aside, sometimes even replacing them with feelings of invulnerability.

But denial can also be a useful tool for coping with the vicissitudes of life. We push aside feelings of rejection by a lover, disappointment at not being offered a desired job, or the reminder that we are overdue for a colonoscopy. At times we use our powers of denial to make life into what we want it to be, not what it actually is.

Denial can be deadly, even more dangerous than depression.

Sometimes denial is even worse than bad medical treatment. A woman with a lump on her breast can choose to ignore it. After all, it may just be a harmless cyst. But if her self-diagnosis of a harmless cyst is wrong and it's a cancerous lump, her denial-enabled waiting has magnified her risk. A delay may result in her eventually needing *more* extensive and difficult-to-tolerate treatments. This waiting game risks making the lump the first step in a fatal disease progression when the result could have been otherwise.

As a person with hemophilia who could suffer grave consequences from playing contact sports or being in a car crash or even tripping and falling, I became a master of denial. With age and experience, my attitude changed. The reality of the nasty bruises, internal bleeding, and even hospitalizations taught me to accept reality and tone down the denial, although I never completely eliminated it.

Facing facts is a key health-care success strategy.

Denial magnifies vulnerability because it permits risky behavior.

As a teenager, I was certain I could play football—after all, it was just "touch" football. But touch football players run into each other; they can be hit in the head by errant throws and tumble to the ground. That can lead to manageable bruises and scrapes for civilians. For me, it caused visits to the emergency room for infusions of clotting-factor drugs. Once, another kid who wasn't sure what touch football meant, pushed me and I fell on my butt. Sitting was incredibly painful for me over the next several months. After decades, that injury I sustained when I was fourteen years old developed into hip-joint arthritis and led to a hip replacement. Most people are not stupid, but we've all made stupid choices.

Bad decisions follow clear patterns. For example, we all tend toward "confirmation bias," in which we recognize only those facts that support the outcome we want to be true. Once you are aware of your susceptibility to it, you can more easily identify it in your own thinking, reject this thinking, and become a clearer independent thinker searching for the best answer. Chapter 7 has more detail on biases that can prevent clear thinking.

During the COVID-19 pandemic, Dr. Anthony Fauci, the former director of the National Institute of Allergy and Infectious Diseases, advised Americans to get vaccinated, wear masks, and stay home. But perhaps you didn't want to do any of those, so you believed online reports by sketchy bloggers about people dying from vaccinations, suffering lung damage from wearing masks, and gaining weight and becoming depressed because they had chosen to follow Dr. Fauci's advice. You ignored and disparaged Dr. Fauci and his guidance.

Another type of poor thinking involves mistakenly ascribing cause and effect. Proving cause and effect in a medical context requires rigorous scientific study with samples that accurately represent the various groups and issues being investigated. This may take years and millions of dollars.

Cause-and-effect thinking may help you raise and explore questions related to your health—for example: Will eating broccoli slow down the growth of my tumor?—but you're best served leaving the conclusions to the experts.

The American All-Star baseball player Joe DiMaggio smoked a cigarette between every inning of every game he ever played. Was this why he was such a great hitter? If you want to impute cause and effect, smoking was the reason he was the best hitter ever.

If you can't think of examples of when you displayed these types of flawed thinking, try harder. Perhaps you wore a copper bracelet as a cure for arthritis, ate raw local honey to control allergies, or used vinegar to cure athlete's foot or irradicate head lice. None of these work. But arthritis, allergies, and athlete's foot are not fatal conditions. Steve Jobs's cancer was dangerous, and he applied similar faulty thinking to his cancer treatment.

If you can identify errors in your thinking, you can avoid these mistakes.

Five Guidelines to Challenge Your Preconceptions, Think Clearly, and Avoid Bad Decisions

1. **Teams make better decisions than individuals.** Don't think that you know better than everyone else. Throughout this book, I stress the importance of team building to support you emotionally and medically. Put that approach to work when facing key treatment decisions and discuss your options with professionals and experienced patients.

2. **"Do-overs" are allowed.** You might choose a doctor you really like, or your uncle recommended, or who validates parking. But after a few weeks, your opinion may become more negative. You can change doctors. You can also change hospitals, group practices, or clinics. Find the doctor best suited to you.

3. **Keep learning.** There is a world of accessible information at your disposal. It takes seven or eight years of intense study to become a doctor after graduating from college. You can't expect to become an expert in your condition after reading a flyer in the doctor's office. There is a huge amount to know, and the reservoir of knowledge keeps growing. Sign up for newsletters from your hospital and the nonprofits that support patients with your condition. Scan the web for podcasts and presentations by reputable sources. Search medical journals and textbooks to narrow the knowledge gap between you and your doctors.

4. **Be skeptical.** As you enter the world of medical treatment, information and guidance will start to come at you from all sides. Take it all in, evaluate it, and look for the few gems that might actually be of help to you in your situation.

5. **Write it down.** Thinking changes when it gets recorded on paper. Of course, it later becomes a record to which you can refer to refresh your memory, but words on paper carry a substance that mere thoughts or memories don't. Documenting your key thoughts and important information can prove invaluable later when making healthcare decisions.

Depression, denial, and poor reasoning feed on feelings of vulnerability and may conspire to keep you out of the medical system. Still, sooner or later, when you can no longer ignore that pain or other symptoms, you will have to enter the health-care system.

The medical system magnifies your perception of this vulnerability. From the moment you enter the building, a hospital reminds you of this. People in wheelchairs, on gurneys, or walking slowly in tandem with an IV pole while dressed in blue hospital robes with their butts hanging out the back are all examples of how hospitals make people feel diminished and vulnerable.

For many patients, the smell of antiseptic is a powerful trigger. It may remind you of visiting your grandmother when she was dying. It may conjure up the time you saw the school nurse when you scraped your knee and she blamed you for not being careful, then wiped your skin with a nasty stinging antiseptic. For me, it brings back painful childhood memories of visits to emergency rooms and long stays in hospital wards.

Many aspects of the medical system can make you feel vulnerable, depressed, frightened, and angry. Being treated rudely, having to wait, or being required to complete the same questionnaire you completed three times before are just some of the many ways the medical system triggers feelings of fear and vulnerability—and, of course, annoyance.

Amid all this seeming chaos, keep in mind that in all likelihood, there is an effective treatment for your scary diagnosis.

After all, you are sitting in that depressing waiting room because you are on a mission to become well and, compared to the importance of that goal, these other issues are trivial.

And then you are finally called to the inner sanctum where the doctor will be . . . But wait, there's more. First you must sit in a cell-like "treatment room" where your vital signs may be measured by a nurse. That takes under a minute. Then you wait, and wait, and wait some more. The door is closed, the room is small and cold.

You are all alone.

Well, just you and your fears.

But remember your mission: to get well.

You are relieved when the doctor arrives. The wait is over, but your fears may ratchet up again. After all, the doctor may give you bad news or no news.

Take a deep breath and remember: this doctor has problems of his or her own. This is not the time for you to be shy or chatty. Doctors are measured by the clock as much as any factory worker. They have likely been told by their administrators that they need to complete a minimum number of *billable* patient interactions—usually six to eight every hour.

You have eight or ten minutes to deal with your issues.

If you think you have hemorrhoids, get to the point—so to speak. If you are embarrassed about parts that are flaccid when they should be firm or firm when they should be flaccid, get over it.

This interaction with the doctor may be productive in curing your problem or minimizing its importance, but don't expect a morale-boosting pep talk. Many doctors don't see giving positive feedback as part of their jobs, nor should you expect it.

Telling you at age sixty that you should plan to live another fifty years—even partially in jest—is not part of medical school education. Congratulating you on losing ten pounds or winning the town bowling tournament are compliments you should look for from your friends, not from your doctor.

The doctor is trained to quickly match problems with solutions—a prescription, the application of an ice pack, or a week of abstaining from sex.

Vague complaints on a doctor's visit—feeling low energy or headaches that come and go—can't be handled in a few minutes, so the physician will likely send you to the lab for bloodwork.

Or they may dispatch you to a specialist. Big or complex issues—everything from insomnia, swollen legs, or consideration of a sex change—earn you a referral to another doctor.

Resign yourself to yet another intake questionnaire that is at least five times as long as the one you just completed or to be sent to yet another specialist.

Three Ways to Prepare for a Doctor's Visit

1. **Make lists.** You can anticipate many of the questions the doctor will ask: What brings you in today? Can you describe the symptoms you are experiencing and how long you have been having them? What medications are you taking? Is there any family history of this problem? Have those answers ready, as well as your own questions for the doctor. Attending these meetings with you and taking notes is also a valuable role for a friend or family member.

2. **Be mission ready.** Keep at the top of your mind that you are there to find answers and solutions, so focus on those. Allowing the conversation to drift into the high prices of real estate or your upcoming college reunion is just wasting the precious few minutes you are being given. *Tick, tock.*

3. **Expect—no, demand—the doctor's full attention.** I once had a doctor's visit interrupted by a call he took from his pool contractor. It was the last time I went to

that doctor. If, for whatever reason, you don't feel you are receiving the physician's full attention, say so. You can do this bluntly: "I really need to have your full attention." Or more subtly: "Perhaps we should find another time to meet."

Don't forget you are a person. You are not a box that needs to be checked.

Just checking in for an overnight or a longer all-inclusive stay at the hospital will familiarize you with the vulnerability machine. First, you are not allowed to walk to your room. You might have run a half marathon, engaged in an hour of sweat-drenched lovemaking, cooked a ten-course meal for your relatives who were wishing you well before you entered the hospital—or even all three activities—and you will still have to sit in a wheelchair, put your bag or possessions on your lap, and let a hospital aide push you to your room.

A hospital in-patient ward is like a factory. But instead of the patients moving down the assembly line, the assembly line of activities moves around them. Aides take vital signs, medical students and interns interview you as part of their required clinical hours for their training, cleaners sweep the floors and check the bathrooms for sloppy patient detritus, and nurses hook you up to IV bags of medicine or fluids and respond, eventually, when the machines beep and demand attention.

The masters of ceremonies are the doctors. But they stop by only for occasional short visits to see how you are doing, report on the latest test results, or update you on when your procedure or surgery is scheduled. And with every patient interaction, the doctor generates a charge to your insurance company. None of these interactions makes you feel like a valued person.

Don't let yourself be dragged down. Entertain yourself.

How can you minimize these feelings of vulnerability or hostility as you enter the belly of the beast? You can't really prevent them. You can only recognize them, be prepared for them, and cope the best you can. In these vulnerable situations, I look around and try to find something humorous or at least ironic.

For example, I find it entertaining how some patients try to discreetly hide their urine sample container as they leave the bathroom. I get a chuckle at the literature that some doctors display in their waiting rooms. They are often about embarrassing conditions, such as plastic surgery options for that double chin, treatments for erectile dysfunction, and weight loss programs.

Hmmm. It seems they were expecting me.

A hospital stay is a break from your regular routine. You may not have been scheduled for a vacation, but being a patient in a hospital should move your focus entirely off work and entirely onto your health. That's not necessarily a bad thing.

Be sure to plan your entertainment before you check in. Bring a book or two that really engage you and will take your mind off worrying. If you have aspired to reach the master's level in Tetris, here's your chance. Bring your phone loaded with games.

Some members of the hospital staff will treat you like a person, engage you in conversation, and make you feel valued as a patient, but others may not. Be prepared.

Chapter 4

SICK CHILDREN

Child patients are different from adult patients. Children develop unique diseases such as pediatric leukemia. Also, when they contract common infectious diseases such as the flu, there can be serious consequences. Kids can also present with genetic disorders such as congenital heart defects—and hemophilia. This chapter presents an overview of the particular and important issues of managing a scary diagnosis with a newborn or young child. I will also share parts of my story about how my disease impacted my childhood, especially my schooling.

Medical treatment of infants and children is both art and science. Their cute little bodies are powerful and efficient at processing everything that goes in, including all manner of drugs from antibiotics to chemotherapy. Children's metabolism is different from that of adults, and some of the rules for treating adults simply don't apply.

As the science of medicine advanced in the eighteenth century, pediatrics was recognized as its own specialty. The first hospital for children opened in Paris in 1802. The first pediatric hospital in the US was Children's Hospital of Philadelphia, which opened in 1855. Treating children has been a growth industry ever since. Today there are over two hundred fifty children's hospitals in the US. Fundraising campaigns for leading children's hospitals, such as St. Jude Children's Research Hospital or Shriners Hospital for Children (now known as Shriners Children), are run nationally in the form of their ubiquitous ad campaigns showing children in wheelchairs or connected to multiple tubes as they lie in beds.

Ava

In many ways, Ava Barron was a typical newborn. She was cute beyond measure, and most times when she opened her eyes from a nap, one or both her parents, Maurice and Kandice, were standing over her bursting with joy that she existed. One morning, when she was thirteen months old, Ava woke up early screaming and vomiting. It was the start of the COVID-19 pandemic, so Maurice and Kandice were concerned, especially as new parents. Their daughter was inconsolable, so they called an ambulance and took Ava to the closest regional hospital with a pediatric emergency room where they lived in New Jersey.

The emergency room doctor's preliminary examination turned up nothing, but the doctor recommended an ultrasound. Then to confirm what the first one showed, he ordered a second scan. This confirmed a tumor on one kidney, and by 7:00 p.m. Ava was admitted to the hospital. Maurice and Kandice's overwhelming joy at being parents in these twelve hours turned into overwhelming fear.

Further tests identified the tumor as a rare and aggressive form of childhood kidney cancer that was fatal more than 90 percent of the time. Memorial Sloan Kettering was one of two hospitals in the world that had extensive experience and some success in treating this type of cancer in infants. Maurice and Kandice decided to have Ava admitted there, and for the next eight months, Memorial Sloan Kettering became their primary home. During her stay, she endured eleven rounds of radiation and eight rounds of chemotherapy. Each treatment wiped out her immune system. Despite heroic efforts with intravenous medications and a gastric feeding tube, Ava's weight fell from twenty-six pounds to twelve pounds. She stopped breathing twice and was resuscitated. She endured five surgeries, including the removal of her cancerous kidney.

Throughout this ordeal, her parents took turns at her bedside. Because of COVID-19 restrictions, only one parent was allowed in the hospital at a time. During the days when she had chemotherapy, Ava was alert and active. But the days after each chemo treatment when her white blood cells and platelet counts plummeted, she became weak and vulnerable.

Ava received blood and platelet transfusions to help bring her energy level back up. The cycle was one week of chemo, two weeks of being incredibly ill, and then a week when her counts came back up. Then the cycle would start all over again.

Throughout the months and regardless of Ava's condition, her parents spoke to her, sang to her, and read her stories. They hoped this would strengthen her connection to them and to life itself.

The physical toll on the parents of a severely ill child is always high, but as the months progressed, the psychological stress on Maurice and Kandice became staggering. Maurice's mood especially deteriorated and he fell into despair. With the hospital visiting policy mandating only parent at a time in the hospital, Maurice and Kandice rarely saw each other. Aside from Ava's fragile condition, she was in a shared intensive care unit in which children were dying, which was incredibly difficult to witness. They worried that Ava might be next.

After Ava's treatments ended, Maurice and Kandice brought her home. Maurice wrote a letter to President Joe Biden. Biden was focused on making improvements in cancer care central to his national health agenda, and Maurice had read President Biden's and Dr. Jill Biden's books on the loss of Biden's son, Beau, to brain cancer. To Maurice's surprise, both President Biden and Dr. Jill Biden responded. President Biden told Maurice that "losing hope would be unforgiveable" and that "you need to steal moments of joy no matter where and when they are." These personal responses from the Bidens helped bolster Ava's parents' spirits.

After eight months of intensive treatment, Ava's cancer went into remission. To bring continuing focus to the president's health agenda, the Bidens invited Ava, Maurice, and Kandice to the White House and to be guests at the president's announcement of his "cancer moonshot" initiative. Ava joined them and participated in the Easter Egg Roll on the White House lawn. The next year, the family was invited back to attend the State of Union speech in February 2023, during which they were to be introduced to the nation from the balcony. But Ava couldn't attend. It was past her bedtime, and she was sound asleep back in the White House.

Today, Maurice's and Kandice's overwhelming fear has been replaced by overwhelming gratitude, and they are finding ways to help other parents cope with their own children's scary diagnoses. They acknowledge that without insurance, access to a top-level hospital, understanding employers, and having loving families and friends, they couldn't have made it through this crisis. Maurice says he simultaneously feels like the unluckiest and luckiest person on earth.

"Why So Much Emphasis on Sick Children?"

There are no fundraising campaigns for treating fat, old men who have spent the last ten years on the couch swilling beer, eating chips, and watching football, despite the fact that this group fills many more hospital beds than sick children. Hospitalization rates track with age: infants are hospitalized the least and older people the most.

So why do we pay so much attention to caring for sick children? Why are there all these hospitals dedicated to pediatrics? Many hospitals have excellent pediatric departments, so why do we need entire hospitals dedicated to the care of children?

Infants and children are different from adults

Indeed, it is dangerous for children to receive treatment from hospitals and doctors who are not pediatric specialists. A recent study by the JAMA Open Network found that over 200 children will die annually after being mistreated in emergency rooms that lacked proper expertise in treating children who had suffered traumatic injuries.

Communication with infants is nonverbal. A neonatologist once explained to me that treating newborns and young infants was like being a veterinarian, interpreting nonverbal cues and communicating through touch, facial expressions, and tone of voice. But once children obtain language skills, medical issues can be explained, they can be reasoned with, and their opinions clearly expressed.

The birth of a child sparks a powerful parenting response that can sometimes be shockingly unexpected. The new baby smell, the perfection of their fingers and toes, and the miracle of a burp connect with some untapped part of new parent brains to trigger a level of love, protectiveness, and connection they have never experienced. If a child becomes sick, parents often experience a level of anxiety and fear beyond what they would experience if they themselves were ill. Seeing or hearing about sick children—even when they are not our own—provokes a similar empathic response. This is what St. Jude and Shriners hospitals tap into when they ask us to donate money.

A key difference between children and adults is that children don't check themselves into hospitals when they feel sick. Someone, usually a parent, has to bring them into the doctor's office or hospital. Psychologists call this a "lack of agency or autonomy." Kids are powerless, but they still require the most intense care and attention of any patient.

As I have discussed, I received this level of care from my parents, especially from my mother. It is only years later—and after becoming a parent—that I was able to appreciate the amount of attention a parent must give to a sick child and the toll this takes on the caregiver. In becoming the parent's top priority, a sick child's needs replace sleep, work, and a social life. It means time spent in doctor's offices, hospitals, and just standing over the crib.

Often the sickest patients in the hospital are the smallest: premature babies. Weighing as little as one pound, with underdeveloped lungs that can't effectively pull oxygen from the air, most seriously premature babies must struggle to overcome daunting odds. Babies born before twenty-five weeks of pregnancy (forty weeks is normal) have only a fifty-fifty chance of living long enough to go home to their families.

Caring for the Youngest and Sickest Patients

Deborah Dokken became pregnant the first time and went into labor after only twenty-five weeks. Her baby girl, Abigail, weighed just under two pounds. Before Deborah or her husband,

Tom, could hold Abigail, she was whisked off to the neonatal intensive care unit (NICU). Abigail would spend the next six months in the NICU and then one week in a pediatric intensive care unit (PICU) before she died.

Abigail did not take this difficult journey alone. Her mother took leave from work so that every day she could sit as close to her daughter as the hospital staff would allow, which sometimes meant sitting next to the incubator or waiting outside the NICU looking in through a window like a visitor in a prison.

Is there any connection between two people stronger than that of a mother and her children? Yet parents of sick children are often relegated to roles as observers. Deborah tells the story of the time a nurse said Abigail could have a bath for the first time. She had been too fragile before. Deborah asked if she could participate with the nurse but wanted to wait fifteen minutes so she could get something to eat from the hospital cafeteria, which was soon closing. The nurse agreed, but when Deborah returned fifteen minutes later, the nurse told her that she had already bathed Abigail. Years later, Deborah still bristles when she tells this story. What is crueler and less considerate of a mother's role than denying her the joy of touching and caring for her baby?

Deborah's story emphasizes the importance of ensuring that the hospital staff respect—indeed appreciate—the unique role that parents play in caring for their child, even when the baby is in the NICU. Today there are organizations, such as the Institute for Patient and Family-Centered Care, which focus on promoting the involvement of family in the care of all patients, especially children. In fact, Deborah is such a strong believer in this mission that she served on their staff for ten years.

Deborah and Tom expressed and endured the grief of Abigail's loss and Deborah became pregnant again. She had surgery to increase the odds of maintaining the pregnancy but their second child, Jonathan, was born after twenty-four weeks and died the same day. The next pregnancy ended in an early miscarriage. Having experienced one miscarriage and the premature loss of two babies, Deborah and Tom knew the risks of another pregnancy were high. They were no strangers to the grief that accompanies pregnancy loss and newborn death. The fortitude to continue after enduring such challenges is as strong a statement of commitment to family as any a couple can make.

For her subsequent pregnancy, Deborah's high-risk specialists recommended a more invasive surgery when Deborah was fourteen weeks pregnant, followed by complete bedrest—first at home and then in the hospital. While Deborah was hospitalized, she also received an experimental treatment to speed up the development of her baby's lungs before birth. After thirty weeks, Jeremy was born. He did well and was able to go home after "only" four weeks in the NICU.

But Deborah's trials as a caregiver were not over. Weeks after Abigail's death, Tom was diagnosed with pseudomyxoma peritonei, an extremely rare cancer that is characterized by the growth of thick mucus-like tumors throughout the abdomen. This led to many difficult surgeries and hospitalizations, including one just ten days after Jeremy's birth and another twenty-hour experimental surgery when Jeremy was only eight months old. Tom lived for twenty-two more years before the doctors decided that no additional surgeries or medical interventions would extend his life.

For Deborah, her husband's death concluded a nearly thirty-year run as a selfless caregiver. I used to wonder if everyone has this capacity or if it surfaces when a person is tested by a scary diagnosis in their family. Now I think that some people have a great gift, like Deborah, to care for others. Those who receive the care they provide are indeed fortunate.

A child's powerlessness may be more painful than their disease. Many of my bleeding episodes that required hospitalizations caused little physical pain. But being confined to a bed, worried about my health and separated from my family and friends, was the worst part of my hospitalizations. This helplessness is obvious to patients, their families and friends, and everyone who watches TV ads soliciting contributions to a children's hospital.

One of the major improvements in pediatric care in recent years is that most pediatric units no longer separate parents from their children. Indeed, most encourage a parent to stay overnight with their child.

Almost everyone has experienced doctors or nurses who are not good listeners and don't seem concerned about their patient's complaints. We don't like it, and we generally blame the provider. Children don't know to do that. When they encounter a doctor or nurse who is condescending or patronizing, they accept this as a statement of reality. A child may well think, "I am less than these people. After all, I am a child and a sick and defective one." All too often, ill children come to experience the world—and themselves—through this lens.

Medical professionals need to provide sick children with the most accurate information, adapted to the age of each child. And they should never lie. Eventually the lie will be revealed and the child will lose trust in the medical system, if not in all adults.

When I was six years old, I asked my mother if I could die from my "condition," which is what we called my hemophilia. She lied and said no. Certainly I put her in a tough spot, confronting her with a question she was not prepared to answer.

In hindsight, saying it was unlikely or that we should ask the doctor on our next visit would have been a better—and more honest—answer.

Sick children are indeed different and special. Their bodies don't follow the rules of adult metabolism, and human empathy for children unlocks resources at all levels to provide specialized care. When medical care for sick children is successful, those children can go on to live long and full lives.

I was one of those special children—born with a genetic disease, rendered powerless by the medical system. But because of continued medical advances in the treatment of hemophilia, I was given a long, full life.

What placed me in this situation was hemophilia, a disease in which blood does not clot properly. The blood-clotting process is a twelve-step ballet of cascading chemical reactions resulting in a clot that plugs up an injury through which blood was leaking or bleeding. Each step has its own unique protein, generally referred to as a clotting factor. Miss one step—or factor—in the process and you don't form a functional clot to properly plug the bleeding. Hemophilia, or the inability to form a clot, most commonly results from missing factor VIII or factor IX. There are rarer types of hemophilia that result from missing other proteins that have their roles in this cascading clotting reaction. According the Centers for Disease Control and Prevention, about 80 percent of people with bleeding disorders are factor VIII deficient, which is referred to as hemophilia A. That's what I inherited. About 10 percent of patients are factor IX deficient, which is called hemophilia B. Another type of hemophilia is von Willebrand disease, named for the Finnish doctor who first identified it in the 1920s, which is caused by a deficiency in a protein aptly called von Willebrand factor.

Hemophilia is usually a genetically inherited disease. Hemophilia A and B are genetically transferred diseases where the faulty gene is located on the X chromosome. If you recall high school biology, you remember that men have one X and one Y chromosome, and women have two X chromosomes. For a man to have hemophilia, he needs the defective gene on his X chromosome. For a woman to have hemophilia, she needs to have defective genes on both of her X chromosomes. As a result, hemophilia A and B are largely diseases of men. Von Willebrand disease is also largely acquired genetically, but it is not linked to gender. About 75 percent of people with hemophilia have a family history of receiving the defective gene from their mother. However, in about 25 percent of cases, there is no family history. This may happen because this gene is in a fragile location on the chromosome and likely to break during cell reproduction, a process called mitosis. Is your high school biology coming back to you?

This X chromosome location of the gene means that women who carry the defective gene on one of their X chromosomes have a 50 percent probability of passing it along to their sons and a 0 percent probability of passing the disease along to their daughters. Their daughters, with one defective gene, will become carriers, 50 percent of their sons will have hemophilia, and 100 percent of their daughters will be carriers. In rare cases of a father with hemophilia and a mother who is a carrier, all their children—both sons and daughters—will have hemophilia.

Even people who don't know much about hemophilia think of it as a royal disease. Queen Victoria was a carrier of hemophilia B. One of her four sons, Prince Leopold, had hemophilia and died at age thirty from a bleed after a fall. Two of her five daughters, Beatrice and Alice, were carriers of the hemophilia gene, and through marriage, spread it to royal houses throughout Europe—most famously to the Russian royal family and to its heir, Tsarevich Alexei Nikolaevich Romanov, the son of Tsar Nicholas II. Alexei's parents were so distraught over his disease that they sought care from the infamous Grigori Rasputin, a mystic and self-styled holy man, who claimed he could treat Alexei through prayer and hypnotism.

Many books and movies have told this story, and Rasputin has become a symbol for medical fakery. As a person with hemophilia, it does, however, seem to me that Rasputin proffered four treatments that might have actually diminished the young Alexei's symptoms. First, Rasputin instructed the royal doctors to leave him alone and let him rest, which is always a good idea with an active bleed. Second, he told the family to stop giving their son aspirin to manage his pain. Aspirin is a powerful anticoagulant and definitely the wrong drug for a person with hemophilia. Third, hypnosis may have actually helped Alexei cope with his pain and sleep better. I have used it myself to good effect. And fourth, Rasputin worked directly with Alexei's distraught mother, Czarina Alexandria, to calm her and reassure her that, although her son could not be cured, his pain could be managed.

But hemophilia is not a disease of royalty. It is spread evenly around the world and among ethnic groups. What is not spread evenly around the world is medical care and access to helpful treatments. Clotting factor drugs, which are state of the art in hemophilia treatment, are not collected from blood but manufactured using recombinant DNA technology in which genetically modified cells create clotting factor in vats like a brewery. In the United States, which is the most expensive market in the world for all drugs, a single adult dose of clotting factor costs around $2,000. It lasts about forty-eight hours before another dose may be required. Most insurance policies cover the cost of clotting factor.

Today, a new generation of treatments is making its appearance through gene therapy. Astoundingly, scientists have harnessed a virus's ability to enter the body's cells and make changes to chromosomes by engineering a denatured virus to carry a healthy version of the gene that controls blood clotting and inserting it in patient's chromosomes. While viruses that alter DNA are generally associated with causing disease, this science turns that process on its head to cure diseases. With the newly corrected gene, patients begin producing their missing clotting factor. Amazing. Gene therapy still needs additional trials to see how well and how long it works and to test for negative side effects. But if it works as hoped, it will be a true cure. One possible glitch: each treatment is likely to cost between $3 and $4 million.

Medical treatment of children generally, and hemophilia specifically, has advanced greatly since my scary diagnosis. My mother was not allowed to stay with me in the hospital, but most hospitals encourage this practice today. When I was a child, there was no one on staff whose job it was to worry about my mental well-being. Today, all children's hospitals and pediatric wards have psychologists, social workers, and child life specialists to mitigate children's medical traumas.

Is it enough? Not really, because not all staff members have been trained to communicate effectively with children. About thirty years after I was a pediatric patient, our two-and-a-half-year-old son had minor surgery. The hospital allowed a parent to stay in the recovery room with him—but only one at a time. My wife and I took turns, but the head nurse wouldn't let one parent in until the other parent had left. This gap of time without a parent made him burst into tears and scream. So, yes, things have become better for young patients, but there will always be room for improvement.

A similar process has taken place in the broader world of schools. Today, schools and families work to mainstream students with disabilities. But this is a rather recent development. Even the idea of working to rehabilitate people with disabilities is less than a century old and received its impetus when President Franklin D. Roosevelt, himself disabled by polio, became an advocate for rehabilitation in the 1930s.

Slowly, over time, the focus on rehabilitation and education grew. Injured World War II veterans organized into an interest group and pressured the government to create rehabilitation programs along with vocational training.

Disability advocates seized the narrative of the 1960s civil rights movement, positioning people with disabilities as a minority group who also received unequal treatment and educational opportunities. This approach was incorporated into the Rehabilitation Act of 1973 that established civil rights for people with disabilities. This was followed in 1975 by the Education for All Handicapped Children Act (EAHCA), which requires public education for children with disabilities and became the foundation of what is today called special education.

In 1990, the Americans with Disabilities Act (ADA) was passed by Congress and ensured that people with disabilities receive equal treatment and access to employment, education, and public accommodations. At the same time, the EAHCA was renamed the Individuals with Disabilities Education Act (IDEA), which codified and reinforced the requirement of access to education for children with disabilities. During this roughly fifty-year span from 1975, the way children with disabilities are managed in public education drastically changed. Today, the general consensus is that although special education accommodations can be expensive, it is the most desirable way to educate and socialize children with disabilities.

My education took place before this movement toward inclusion. At that time, students with disabilities were segregated into their own classes that had low or no standards and were often seen as babysitting services.

My parents did not want me put in that group, so they lied. Until I started the seventh grade, they asked my pediatrician for notes saying that I couldn't participate in physical activities but could attend academic classes. I was told to say that I had an injured ankle—which was true—and that prevented me from taking gym classes—which was a lie.

I spent many hours sitting on the sidelines or staying in an empty classroom while the rest of the class had gym. But to my parents' credit, their strategy was the best option. I took classes with the mainstream students, did well, and advanced academically and socially in my education. Was it a perfect solution? Hardly! I felt isolated and lonely, and saw myself as physically defective.

Yet the alternative would have been placing me with severely disabled children and poorly trained teachers in a setting in which learning was minimal. I see now that my experience was early evidence of the value of mainstreaming students with physical disabilities to the greatest extent possible.

Of course there is a wide variety of disabilities and illnesses that interfere with mainstreaming students. Some students require tutoring by teachers trained in understanding and educating children with various disabilities. Others require only enough classroom space to park a wheelchair.

Guidelines for Managing Illness in Children

- Children are not just small adults. They are unique physically and mentally.
- Seek treatment at hospitals that are recognized for and highly ranked in pediatrics.
- Children are smart and perceptive. Don't lie to them. Give them as much truth as they can understand.
- Manage a sick child's health so that he or she can live in the mainstream.
- Provide care to the entire family, not just the sick child.

Chapter 5
BUILDING YOUR TEAM

We live our lives in teams: the sales team at work, a bowling team, the committee that organizes the street fair in your neighborhood, and, of course, your family. Two reasons that teams exist: First, many activities simply can't be accomplished by an individual, such as playing a string quartet or a game of baseball. Second, delegating tasks to different team members allows each person to focus on their expertise and raise the overall quality of the work the team produces.

Exposure to the medical system and interaction with sick friends and family members impacts individuals very differently. Some people have strong emotional reactions, while others have little response or suppress their feelings. At an early age, I began to appreciate the delegation of work to different family members. My father worked long hours in his deli, so my mother took the lead on my care, sometimes with the help of other relatives. But together they formed my health-care team.

My mother took me to all my doctors' appointments and hospital visits, enforced the doctors' rules, and worked directly with my teachers when I missed so much school that I was behind on my assignments. She was always the one urging caution and fearful of any risky actions by me that might cause a bleed. When I began school, Mom would drop me off, return home, and climb back into bed. I would later learn that she was so fearful of my being hurt at school that she would try to sleep through those hours until I came home.

My father worked long hours in his deli and directly managed little of my health-care regimen. The first time he visited me in the hospital, watching his son receive a blood transfusion overwhelmed him. He never visited me in the hospital again.

But Dad took on other responsibilities by seeing that his sick son was able to live a relatively normal life. When the doctors prescribed a bland diet, lest it trigger further intestinal bleeding, Dad took me for Italian food and encouraged me to try the spicy items. "Don't tell your mother," he said. At a local fair in the New Jersey town where we had a summer house, he entered us in the three-legged race, which was fun but enraged my mother. To this day, I don't know if he was encouraging these activities because he thought it was good for me to experience a more normal childhood or good for him to feel his son was not as fragile as his wife feared.

Dad took me to sporting events, brought me on long walks through New York neighborhoods, introduced me to exotic foods, and to the extent possible, gently tried to teach me sports. He had been a serious athlete—a runner and a baseball player—and perhaps he wanted his son to be as much like him as possible. But I have come to believe that his encouragement was good for me, enabling me to prove that I had some physical capacities and physical activity could bring me joy. This was a welcome antidote to the hours spent sitting alone at school while the rest of the class had gym.

My older brother, who didn't have hemophilia, also let me tag along with some of his activities, such as going to folk music concerts and shooting baskets at the playground. Baseball was played with a soft rubber ball, and football was reduced to a game of catch. My brushes with this normality were delicious beyond description.

I can't fathom how anyone could cope with a serious medical issue alone. From management of one's medications to transportation to doctors' offices to emotional support, there are essential roles for team members to play.

As an adult, I became largely self-sufficient in my health care. When I turned twenty, the clotting factor that I kept at home in my refrigerator and self-infused became the standard of care and main treatment modality for nearly forty years.

When I was fifty-nine, it became clear that my liver was failing from the effects of hepatitis C and I needed a liver transplant. After being largely self-sufficient in my care, the overwhelming importance of a highly involved partner became crucial. There are so many appointments and judgments to make about health-care professionals and potential treatments that required conversation and consultation with someone I loved and trusted. No one can provide this more than the person whose face you see across the pillows at the beginning and end of each day.

My friend and fellow professor Don Schepers, who was diagnosed with Parkinson's disease when he was sixty-one years old, sees his support network as a set of different spheres. The most central sphere consists of his wife, Jeanne, who is one of the most caring and loving people I have ever known. Don says, "I experience absolute support from her. She is constantly checking to make sure I am okay, particularly when she has to leave me for a period of time." Jeanne's support also has a dimension of pushing Don to go past his limitations to exercise, play golf, and socialize with family and friends. In other words, encouraging Don to maintain as normal a life as possible.

Don and his medical team also include Jeanne as an active participant in his care. She attends every visit with the neurologist and neurotherapist, which his doctors encourage because they need her firsthand assessments of Don's health.

The secondary sphere of Don's support network comprises the neurologist, who does an annual assessment, and his neurotherapist, who consults with Don in person several times a year. To foster easy contact, both of these key members of his medical team encourage the use of email as necessary. Don also lists his brothers and their families as part of the secondary sphere. "They have all been very considerate in making sure we are included in events, and they invite us out from time to time," he explains. "My brothers have also been very generous in helping with projects around the house that I can no longer manage on my own."

Don is still active outside the house, including meeting with a group of retirees twice a week for breakfast and to gab (the proverbial McDonald's group of old guys), and he has made friends through his church. Don counts those two groups as his third sphere.

Don is candid about managing his Parkinson's. He notes, "If I had to do this alone, I would be very frightened. Even with the best medical support, it would be very trying given all the potential complications (falls, choking, inability to communicate, hallucinations, delusions, dementia, and much more). Maybe the uber-rich can afford the amount of care required, but money only goes so far. A true companion is priceless."

When my wife and I became friends with Don and Jeanne, they were foster parents to babies, many of whom had disabilities. They didn't have children of their own, and over six years this rotating group of infants in need had become their family. Even after the babies were given permanent homes, Don and Jeanne kept in touch with them. Some of these newly formed families even come and visit this warm and open couple who gave their babies a loving start in life.

In a rather astounding way, the well-being of these foster children has become Don and Jeanne's North Star—providing a clear focus on what is most important in life. In fact, the day Don received his diagnosis, they were providing foster care to a baby I'll call Nick, who had Down syndrome and club feet. Don said, "One of my first thoughts was that I had sixty-one years of excellent health. With this child in my arms, who was I to complain, to do a 'Woe is me' over my condition? This felt like a moment of true grace, and I've tried to hold on to that throughout." Nick, now eleven, has learned to walk and speak, and attends school. Don says that "the joy and reality children have brought to our lives is irreplaceable and constantly remind me of the gift of life."

Who Will Be Members of Your Team?

Here are the roles that need filling:

Caregiver. Caregivers go with you to medical appointments, and perform or arrange for other help such as cleaning services, home nursing, or shopping. Because of the significant amount of time that you may spend with a caregiver, it is essential to choose one with whom you feel very comfortable.

The Amateur MD. The amateur MD is someone who is knowledgeable and experienced in health care and medicine with whom you can discuss the options your doctors have presented. This might be a friend who is a social worker who has worked with patients and families in similar situations to yours or a relative who is a retired nurse who has years of experience with the medical system.

Bureaucracy Wrangler. Sooner or later, you are going to run into frustrations with the medical bureaucracies. It might be the insurance company, the hospital, or a medical practice. Straightening out the red tape requires time spent on hold, patience beyond measure, and a strong sense of moral indignation to be motivated to be your best advocate.

Buddy. Being alone is one of the most difficult parts of being sick at home or in the hospital. You need the support of people you simply enjoy being with. Perhaps they are friends you like to hear talk about their lives, or people with whom you like to chat about the news. You love being with them, and they keep loneliness at bay.

Masters of Fun. Some friends may not have lots of time to give you but being with them boosts your spirits and brings the real world to you in fun and engaging ways. Perhaps they pick up food from a favorite restaurant or organize a small group to visit you and play board games. When they leave, you may be tired but smiling.

Therapist. As you cope with your scary diagnosis, you can't keep all your thoughts, hopes, and fears to yourself. A well-trained, professional therapist might be best, but a wise friend who is an especially good listener can also serve this role.

Chief Financial Officer. No matter your medical issues, bills still need to be paid, insurance forms completed, and financial planning examined. Perhaps you have an especially trustworthy friend who is a lawyer or an accountant who will be willing to help.

These roles can be filled by one or more people, by family members or friends, or by people you pay. The key is to choose reliable and capable people who put your interests first. If you have trouble filling out your team, contact the hospital social work department, which will have resources to help you and will likely also sponsor patient support groups you can join.

Team Members You Should Avoid

As well-meaning as most people are, there are some friends and family who do more harm than good and should be moved off your team:

The Pity Partygoers. Some friends and relatives just seemed wired to see the world through a negative lens. I have had friends tell me "how sorry they are for me." I don't want to hear this. Please just be caring and loving. Pity is minimizing and debilitating. It is a pessimistic view of the world, and having that attitude does nothing to help support my recovery.

Self-Declared Nobel Prize–Winning Experts. Some friends and family dispense medical advice and then insist that you follow it. After all, they had a great experience with a certain doctor, so everyone should see this doctor. These decisions are yours. Being pressured by people you may care about but who have little true knowledge is aggravating.

Former Friends. Some people just don't want to be around sick people. I understand. I don't want to be around sick people or be the sick person myself. But this is not something about which true friends have a choice. When my father became ill, I witnessed two types of family and friends: those who drew closer, visited and called regularly, and were genuinely concerned about his condition; and those who withdrew, making few visits and otherwise expressing little concern for him. The first group is valuable beyond measure. The second group are now only a part of your past, not your present or future.

Chapter 6

YOU MUST NEVER LOSE YOUR DIGNITY

All of us want and expect to be treated with respect, yet sometimes it seems as if illness and the health-care system have developed ultra-efficient ways to deprive us of our dignity. For many patients feeling vulnerable after hearing their scary diagnosis, losing their dignity is devastating.

As I have discussed throughout this book, being a patient often requires that you manage much of the process—insurance, appointments, family issues, treatments, medications, and more—by yourself. But you also need to manage the medical system to ensure that it treats you respectfully. Keeping you waiting, talking to you as if you understand very little, or not actively engaging you in key decisions are all examples of how the system can make you feel diminished. Let's talk about how you can prevent losing your human dignity.

Make it clear to caregivers that you are to be treated respectfully. When a nurse's aide in a clinic called me "sweetheart," I found it patronizing and I told her not to do that. When waiting times became extreme, I asked my doctors how they liked being kept waiting for long periods of time. While these conversations may be uncomfortable, if you don't have them, your dignity can be chipped away. Being active and candid about the smaller issues will head off the bigger ones.

Courtesy and respect are two-way streets. Doing your best to be pleasant and respectful to your caregivers signals a partnership. Treating others with respect signals that you also want to be treated with respect. While these issues may not rise to the level of caring for your emotional needs, you cannot expect staff to cater to you and take care of your emotions when you are treating them like servants—and vice versa.

If you feel that you are being treated in a way that threatens your dignity, confront the person responsible and demand that it stop. If the staff member won't listen to you, speak with a supervisor or a patient advocate (a staff position in most hospitals)—or even the president of the hospital. Do whatever it takes to stand up for yourself.

My first two childhood hospitalizations scarred me for life. Instead of making me recognize my right to dignity, the medical staff made me feel insignificant and worthless—feelings that even today can be triggered by negative interactions with others in almost any context. These early hospital experiences were the worst days of my life. Unfortunately, like many people who go through dreadful and painful moments, I never spoke of these experiences to family or friends. But the memory of these experiences and the emotions they trigger can never be erased.

At five years old, I had never spent a night away from home or without my parents and older brother. Peeing red qualified me for hospital admission the first time, and pooping red qualified me for the second. By that point I had lost a great deal of blood.

The treatment in the 1950s for adding clotting factor to my blood was through transfusions of whole blood. Until I was a teenager, and more concentrated forms of clotting factor had been distilled, plasma transfusions were the state-of-the-art treatment. Plasma is the liquid part of blood that remains when the blood cells are removed; it is also where the clotting factor that my blood needed resides.

The underlying problem with plasma treatment is the math. An adult has about five quarts of blood. As a child, I probably had about three quarts of blood, of which about half—around three pints—was plasma. It would be simple to transfuse a full amount of plasma to provide my blood with a normal level of clotting factor, but the body can't process that much additional fluid in the circulatory system quickly enough. Transfuse too much fluid and serious complications, even death, can result. I received one unit (one pint) of plasma per day, which took from thirty minutes to an hour to drip slowly into one of my veins. While this never brought me up to the normal level of clotting factor that would stop whatever bleeding was going on, it helped.

These episodes of internal bleeding took place during medically ancient times. The butterfly needles that we are all familiar with today didn't exist. Today, when a long-term intravenous infusion is set up, a needle with a flexible plastic tube inside is used. After it is inserted, the metal tube that is the "needle" is withdrawn, the plastic tube stays in the vein, and the patients retain mobility of their arms.

When I was hospitalized as a child, the metal needle was all there was, and it had to be left in my vein with my arm immobilized by taping it to a board that ran from my wrist to my shoulder.

As a result, my arm would ache or go numb. I couldn't get out of bed, and the tape that covered my entire arm was painful to remove. Often my arm would stay on the board for a week. When the board was removed, it would take another day or two for my arm to regain feeling and mobility. After a week of lying down, I would have to sit for an hour before I was able to stand up without being dizzy.

The first night of my first hospitalization, I was put in one of six beds in a pediatric ward with each bed separated by a high glass barrier embedded with a tightly twisted wire mesh that formed a repeating hexagonal pattern. To me, it looked like a barbed-wire wall. Having spent hours staring at it, I can see it clearly today. It became a symbol of my captivity. In fact, when I see hexagons today, whether in bathroom tiles or the pavers on the main paths at Columbia University, those glass dividers are the first image that comes to mind, along with the feeling of captivity they triggered.

My mother was permitted to stay with me until visiting hours ended at 4:00 p.m. When she was told she had to leave, she asked—begged actually—to stay with me, but in a 1950s pediatric ward, the rules were the rules.

For the first time in my life, I was alone, away from my family.

My five roommates were a varied group. Two had rigid IV lines like mine; the three others did not. Two were very quiet, while the other three were jumping around and making a racket between scoldings from the nurse. I was terrified and don't recall saying a word to anyone. I suppose we were fed; I can't remember. I do recall the urinal hanging on the rail of the bed for me to fill with red pee.

As night came, the hospital floor became quiet, as did my roommates. The lights were turned out. Through my hexagonal wire glass and the door to the ward, I could see a nurse's aide sitting at a desk with a television in front of her. There were rabbit-ear antennae on top, reaching out for signals. I couldn't sleep and became more and more anxious. As an excuse for human contact, I called out several times, asking the nurse's aide what time it was until, with venom in her voice, she told me not to ask her again. Perhaps I was interrupting *The Tonight Show*.

In the middle of the night, a nurse came in and my second dose of plasma was started. As I would do for many hours in the coming years, I watched the yellow-orange plasma drip from the bag, first into a little reservoir and then run into the clear tube down through the needle into my arm. Unable to move, unable to engage anyone in conversation, and far removed from my family, I became more terrified and anxious. My roommates were asleep, the nurse hated me, and in these dark ages, there was no call button on the bed. I was out of options.

I turned to God. My family was somewhat religious, so prayer was familiar to me. My mother had taught me how to pray every night before going to bed. So, from the dark pit of my fear and anxiety, I prayed to God, asking that my loneliness, terror, panic, and discomfort be relieved. I was not reaching out to a theoretical god. I was speaking to a real God. Then God answered. I began to feel warm and itchy. My skin became covered in patches of red, irritated skin. Then those patches raised up in anger.

God had answered me with hives, and the hives brought a battalion of care providers and the attention I was craving!

I interrupted *The Tonight Show*, showed the nurse the hives, and soon my bed was surrounded by the medical professionals.

The doctors looked here and there, poked in places, asked me if I had ever had this before (no), and prescribed a shot of something. In hindsight, it was almost certainly Benadryl, which is an effective and powerful antihistamine to suppress allergic reactions. In ten minutes, my hives were receding. But more importantly, Benadryl makes people sleepy. It knocked me out until I awoke the next morning with my mother standing next to the bed. God had indeed answered this five-year-old's prayer.

About a year later, I developed an intestinal bleed, and the treatment regimen was repeated. I was taken to the same ward with the same twisted hexagonal-wire reinforced glass dividers. One of the ward's previous inmates was still there. My arm was taped to a board, the IV needle inserted, and the plasma started to drip in again. Even the night nurse's aide and her TV were the same. But I was more relaxed. I suppose being a veteran at this—being a year older, and knowing that God would answer my prayers—calmed me. The regular doses of Benadryl that accompanied every bag of plasma helped, too.

After a week I was not better, and I was told that the IV had to be moved to my other arm. The plan was to remove the needle, rip off the tape, and release the arm from the board. Then the same process of taping my other arm down and starting an IV was repeated. But one week was about all I could take, and I was very upset at the prospect of adding another week shackled to the bed.

The doctors didn't talk to me—they *literally* did not talk to me about my condition or how much longer I would have to remain in the hospital. I understand that I was only six years old, but I was still a person.

They didn't see it that way.

I told the doctors that I would *not* submit to having another IV put in until I knew when I would be able to go home. Perhaps this was not a reasonable demand, but this was precisely what was on my mind. And it was a subject the doctors could, at least, address.

They refused. Instead, they told me that if I didn't cooperate, they would restrain me and put in the IV. They did both.

They rounded up a posse of staff, moved my bed to a treatment room, and shifted me onto a cold steel table. I was screaming and flailing, but I was no match for the eight or ten arms that held me down, taped my arm to a board, and inserted the IV needle for next week's plasma. I remember the room, the white subway tiles on the wall, the small window high above the table I was held to, and the doctors and nurses who refused to talk to me.

Even today, more than sixty years later, I can't tolerate doctors who won't engage with me as a person. I can't even imagine doctors treating a child like this. I can't watch movies in which children are mistreated; I become claustrophobic in small spaces, and I don't like white subway tiles.

I suppose this is how to give a six-year-old post-traumatic stress disorder. It only took about ten minutes.

As horrible as these two experiences were—and still are for me to recollect—they changed me and taught me a lesson I have never forgotten. While they may have prematurely ended my childhood and innocence, they taught me a fundamental lesson of personal resilience, showing me that I possessed the ability to cope with what the world was flinging at me.

More than fifty years later, while going through my liver transplant, I often reminded myself that if I could cope with the terrifying circumstances I endured as a five- and six-year-old, I could marshal that same inner strength to cope with receiving a transplant.

If you are feeling sorry for me, don't. It's not my intention. Pity diminishes the recipient, rather like interactions with the health-care system do. Yes, I went through horrible crises, but I made it through them and am tougher for it.

When you find yourself coping with your scary diagnosis, it may well trigger memories of previous negative experiences you have had.

But you made it through them, learned from them, and are tougher because of them. These experiences, like mine, have shown you the resilience and inner strength that you possess but perhaps never had to muster.

Three Tools to Maintain Your Dignity

1. **Don't allow the system to ignore your comfort.** When a parent lovingly tucks their child into bed, they are sending a message to their child that he or she is precious. Having your comfort ignored by a nurse's aide who won't change sweat-soaked sheets sends exactly the opposite message. Speak up.

2. **Maintain human contact with others.** The worst punishment a prisoner can experience is solitary confinement. A bed in a private room or a bed in an intensive care ward both feel pretty close to solitary confinement. To whatever extent you can, seek engagement with others. Having a roommate may be annoying at times, but, on the whole, it will reduce that feeling of isolation.

3. **Stay connected to family and friends.** Our key relationships define us. Don't neglect them or let them be taken away. Reach out to others. Even if visits are not possible, you can always stay in touch with phone or video calls.

Chapter 7

DISTRUST AND SUSPICION

My parents were typical of their generation—they saw doctors as gods. They never questioned a doctor's diagnosis or treatment plan. Obtaining a second opinion was never even considered. That was then.

Subsequent generations have come to have more complex—and less trusting—relationships with doctors. Today we see ads promoting drugs and telling us to "ask your doctor about." The internet answers many of our medical questions within seconds. Some of it is right, much of it is wrong, and almost all of it is designed to sell us something. By the time many people see a doctor, they believe they already know their diagnosis and their treatment options.

The problem is that our attitudes, beliefs, fears, and even knowledge can interfere with the process of finding the correct diagnosis and treatment. Our biases and prejudices underlie and sometimes dominate our thinking, even as we may not even acknowledge they exist. The Nobel Prize–winning economist Daniel Kahneman studied the differences between fast and slow thinking, concluded that many decisions are conditioned by habits and what we have learned from others. (Daniel Kahneman, *Thinking Fast and Slow*, Farrar, Straus and Giroux, 2011.) While we may think we are acting rationally, research like this proves otherwise.

Upon hearing a scary diagnosis, your chances of making bad decisions are high. Accepting the limitations of your thinking, whether because of bias or emotional issues, requires humility and will lead you to better decision-making.

My goal in this chapter is to present the common mistakes that we make in dealing with medical issues so that you can avoid them and be ready to approach your scary diagnosis in the most productive way.

Like most people, I am a person of profound biases and prejudices. And like most people, some of my biases are based on fact and help me make good decisions. For example, I am prejudiced against doctors who take calls from their swimming pool contractors during an exploration of my prostate gland. Yes, it happened. I have a strong bias against doctors whose offices look like pharmacy storage rooms; it makes me wonder whom they are working for. I have a strong bias against doctors—and here I will include dentists—who chronically run late and then tell me they had to deal with an emergency. Really? Maybe occasionally, but not before every one of my appointments. I have a bias against doctors who don't make eye contact with me. I know the computer requires their input, and I know that their smartphone is constantly receiving text messages about tonight's dinner plans, but I want to be their main focus when we meet in person, via video call, or by phone.

But many biases and prejudices represent poor and faulty thinking that interferes with a patient's ability to make good health-care decisions. When we have strong biases about health care, the discussion in our heads is about confirming prejudices and not about what we should do to get better. If we believe that doctors overprescribe drugs or are too eager to perform surgery, our exploration of the medical system may confirm our beliefs by finding doctors who will agree with us—and we will not necessarily obtain the correct diagnosis or the best treatment. A psychologist would call this *confirmation bias*.

You almost certainly know of someone who delayed care for far too long. My friend Harriett hated going to doctors. Only great discomfort, such as a urinary tract infection or a fractured bone in her foot, would force her to overcome her reluctance. But why this reluctance? Harriett was a bundle of fears and biases. She was afraid that the doctor would find "something serious." She didn't like being semi-disrobed in front of strangers. She had a bias against doctors, feeling they were only motivated by money. Harriett's mother had died of colon cancer, and her father of heart disease. While these facts motivate unbiased patients to prevent these diseases from becoming their health futures, they were not enough to overcome her bias. When she finally scheduled a long-delayed colonoscopy, she couldn't tolerate the vile prep drink and canceled the test. I knew her well and believe that her biases against doctors kept her from obtaining preventative care.

We all have some fundamental types of bias and prejudice to some degree, but when they overwhelm reasoned thought, they can become problematic.

Be Honest—Do You Have Any of the Following Biases?

- **Attribution bias** exists when someone—without evidence—attributes a cause or motivation to observed behavior. For example, believing that the doctor wants to do surgery for financial gain. When you have no evidence of this motivation, you are displaying attribution bias, and this bias may become a reason or excuse for delaying or passing on necessary surgery.

- **Confirmation bias** is similar to attribution bias but is based on long-held views. For example, if you continue to believe that emotional stress is the main cause of heart disease, despite evidence that high blood pressure, high cholesterol, and smoking are far more responsible, you are employing confirmation bias. A patient with this bias may dismiss a diagnosis of elevated blood pressure and simply attribute their cardiovascular issues to current stress at work, thus avoiding effective and necessary treatment.

- **Cognitive dissonance** exists when we hold two conflicting ideas and feel a need to reconcile them. For example, we know colon cancer is bad but hate the idea of someone putting a six-foot hose up our butts. So we may conclude that some medical tests are unnecessary, reconciling our fear of the treatment with fear of the potential diagnosis.

- **Prejudice** is having any opinion without evidence. Being prejudiced against people based on race, gender, age, religion, or body weight are all common examples. Prejudiced patients will allow stereotypes to replace clear thinking. I have a friend whose mother would only see doctors with offices in Manhattan. According to her, there were no good doctors in Brooklyn.

The key point for someone who has received a scary diagnosis is that individual biases and prejudices can interfere with obtaining the most accurate diagnosis and making the best decisions to receive the most effective care. Here are descriptions of some common types of patients who let their biases and prejudices interfere with obtaining the best care. Do you recognize any of these traits?

- **Shoppers.** These patients seek advice from doctors, friends, other patients, family members, and even astrologers. Hearing many different conflicting views, they use this as an excuse to do nothing. Or they may shop until they find a doctor who confirms their biases by telling them what they want to hear.

- **Amateur Physicians.** Who needs doctors when you can read everything on the internet and reach your own conclusions? These patients learn to have professional-level discussions with their doctors, but all they really want is to confirm their "medical expertise."

- **Avoiders/Deniers.** Like Harriett, some people who accept the general value of tests or treatment still fear being in the medical system and avoid it by denying that they need any tests or treatment. They will tell you that they expect to live as long as their great-grandmother who smoked three packs a day, never went to a doctor, and lived to a hundred.

- **Buddies.** Some patients mistake friendliness and chattiness for competence, care, and concern. My mother had a gerontologist buddy, and after waiting over an hour to see her, my mother would tell me about the doctor's family, her trips, and her struggles to lose weight. The doctor needed a therapist, and my mother needed a better doctor.

- **Munchausen Syndrome.** This disease describes people who invent conditions or self-inflict symptoms that require medical evaluation and treatment because they want attention. There are documented patients with Munchausen who were so successful at fooling doctors that they received unnecessary tests and even surgeries. A variant is Munchausen syndrome by proxy in which a person projects or actually inflicts health issues onto someone in their care, such as a child or parent. Fortunately, they are rare birds.

When dealing with your scary diagnosis, strive to be a clear thinker. This isn't easy. When I was told that I needed a liver transplant and had perhaps a year to live without one, my mind went to thinking about how to spend that year rather than focusing on how to obtain a transplant. It took me a few weeks to get my priorities in order. Many beliefs and fears in our brains derail clear thinking. The fight-flight-freeze response, in which thinking stops but high hormone levels take over and one of these automatic responses takes place, is a common reaction to great stress. Trying to limit these reactions in order to maintain perspective on your emotions and thinking is a tremendous benefit to good decision-making.

In my experience, these three guidelines help:

1. **Being suspicious is good.** Being paranoid is bad. Not everyone you will encounter in the health-care system is great at what they do, and some won't put your interests first. Being suspicious and questioning helps avoid working with or being treated by the wrong doctors. But becoming paranoid and trusting no one is not the answer. I truly believe that most people in the health-care system are well-intentioned and primarily motivated to do their best for you. Don't suspend your judgment if

you encounter the few who aren't. Instead, welcome the large majority who are sincere about helping you.

2. **Being cautious is good.** Being distrustful is bad. You don't want to jump at the first offer to perform major surgery or be entered in an experimental drug trial. These decisions need to be reviewed, evaluated, and perhaps become part of seeking a second opinion. Being distrustful of every option may cause you to make mistakes and miss important options.

3. **You need others to go through the system with you.** There is simply too much information for most people to process—especially if you are ill and afraid. Friends or family members who will form a team around you can bring clear thinking, flag and help you move beyond biases, and become your trusted advocates.

Chapter 8

SELECTING AND MANAGING YOUR DOCTOR

Doctors are the centerpiece of the health-care system. In large part, they have designed it, written its rules, and lobbied the government to support it financially; and through doctor-friendly regulation, they are its main financial beneficiaries. Of course, drug and insurance companies haven't done so bad either. For most patients, their doctor is not just the centerpiece of a huge system but they also represent the entire health-care system. As a result, choosing the right doctor is critical to your health.

In today's health-care system, you may have little input into selecting your doctor since your insurance company may dictate your options. You are also limited by location and your ability to obtain an appointment.

But you still have agency and you should use it. Don't hesitate to offer your input.

Choosing a doctor is like hiring someone in a business.
There is a job description, an organization to work in, and customers. You are the customer, and your opinion should matter the most. An experienced human resource manager once told me that he hired people based on a "chemistry test." He explained that while he considered qualifications, experience, the opinions of others, he relied more on his gut feeling about how well he could work with this person. That's the chemistry test, and you can try it with doctors you are considering "hiring" to join your team.

Perhaps a friend or relative may have offered you a suggestion for a physician to see, or a doctor you use and like may have recommended a professional colleague. Most doctors haven't been patients of the physicians they recommend, so they may not know if these doctors relate to their patients as people. There is probably little about the recommendation that is actually related to the qualifications of the doctor or to how they relate to their patients as people.

If you think your internist or another doctor can make a judgment about these issues, you might want to think again. It is unlikely your internist tracked the treatments provided to patients by the doctor they recommended to you. And just because the doctor they recommend was personable to them does not mean that same doctor will be understanding and considerate with you.

However, relying on a recommendation may be the best you can do, and I've had some referrals work out wonderfully. Below and in a later chapter, I offer more specific guidance on finding a doctor, including managing insurance restrictions, judging the source of the recommendation, and coping with information you find online. Unsurprisingly, the search can be challenging.

More doctors have put their cold stethoscopes on me than I can count. About a dozen became my care providers over many years. Some became friends. Most were quite good. A few, not good. Let me tell you about the bad ones first.

When I was young and there was little effective treatment for hemophilia, I had a progression of doctors who mainly urged my parents to keep me from being injured and hope for the best. The net effect of this approach was to make my parents anxious and me resentful of them for trying to restrict my activities.

The doctors I saw only one or two times were generally ignorant about hemophilia. They asked me questions that revealed their lack of knowledge about my genetic disease. For example, "How did you catch hemophilia?" "Do you worry much about bleeding from paper cuts?"

I'm not making these comments up. I can't blame them. Most doctors—who are not hematologists—can go their entire careers without ever seeing a patient with hemophilia.

But there is a group of doctors that we all should be highly critical of: the self-interested doctors who put their needs and issues above those of their patients. Some are financially focused—such as the hepatologist I saw when I first contracted hepatitis C as a teenager. At the time, hepatitis C didn't even have a name. It was referred to as "non-A, non-B hepatitis."

In other words, it was called "we have no friggin' idea." There was no effective treatment. Nonetheless, its effects showed up on liver enzyme tests as the liver struggled to rid itself of this once unknown and unnamed virus.

With no treatment to offer, this doctor nevertheless made me come to his office for bloodwork every week for months. These tests added nothing to his knowledge and had no impact whatsoever on my treatment—because there was no treatment.

I was naïve and ignorant, but eventually I realized that I was a cash cow (bleeding cow?) for him. This doctor ran the tests in his private office, away from the hospital, on his own testing equipment, which allowed him to bill the insurance company directly and keep all the revenue. He still failed to devise a treatment plan.

Becoming a doctor solely for the financial rewards is a bad idea. Yes, they have sacrificed through years of school and training. Yes, many have taken on mountains of debt. Yes, they want comfortable lives for themselves and their families. But if they lose sight of their mission as doctors, patients will suffer under their care.

Fortunately, despite the negatives, many doctors never disconnect from their desire to help people and achieve great personal satisfaction doing just that. These are the physicians you need to find, and I believe the chemistry test I just described will do more to identify them than anything else.

When I became an adult and as hemophilia care advanced through the development of clotting factor concentrates, my care moved to comprehensive hemophilia treatment centers, which offered a variety of specialists under one roof. This was—and is—a terrific way to provide care to patients with complex issues. When my liver disease was discovered, my care moved to liver specialists—that is, hepatologists—and to the transplant center that provided comprehensive care to its patients awaiting or recovering from transplants.

Since 2002, Dr. Christopher Walsh has been the chief physician of the Hemophilia Treatment Center at Mount Sinai Hospital in New York City. Dr. Walsh holds an MD and a PhD, which means he both enjoys science and wants to help people. During his tenure, an increased understanding of the chemistry and genetics of hemophilia resulted in an evolution in treatment, including gene therapies that are actual cures. Managing these treatments is complex and requires a doctor who truly understands the science. Having worked with people in various fields from sports to physics, I can attest that only some of them have both truly mastered their subjects and can explain them in simple, clear terms. These qualities describe Dr. Walsh. He is an expert in genetic treatments and explains the medical issues to his patients and their families in clear and understandable language. Unfortunately, when I needed to begin treatment for hepatitis, I had to change doctors.

This process of trying new doctors was not new to me, and it reminded me of early warning signs that I had previously experienced—doctors who chronically run late, hand out drug samples like candy, spend precious time talking about their interests such as golf or travel, or encourage patients to try untested drug regimens. In all these cases, they are putting themselves ahead of their patients. The liver specialists at New York Hospital were in the forefront of new treatments for hepatitis C, so I left Mount Sinai for what I hoped would be the best treatment available.

When I arrived at New York Hospital, the staff immediately ordered an MRI for a good look at my liver. The look was good, but the liver was not. They gave me the bad news and told me to make an appointment with their transplant center. I alerted Dr. Walsh, and he told me that I should come back to Mount Sinai to see hepatologist Dr. Leona Kim-Schluger. He gave her the strongest positive recommendation, which I trusted.

A week later, I had my first meeting with Dr. Kim-Schluger. She had already studied the MRI from the other hospital and agreed that a new liver was in order. She wanted to start the process of placing me on the list at Mount Sinai to be considered for a transplant, but because the waiting list for transplants was so long in New York City, she also recommended that I contact transplant centers at other hospitals.

After speaking with Dr. Kim for three minutes, I felt that I had a good idea of the type of person she is: brilliant and hardworking. I imagined that from the first grade through medical school she never received a grade below A. She impressed me as someone who became a doctor because studying medicine was intellectually challenging and full of questions that are often not easy to answer. To my benefit, Dr. Kim was answering my questions with the information I needed to hear.

As our first meeting wrapped up, I told Dr. Kim that I would thank Dr. Walsh for the introduction, adding that Dr. Walsh was the best doctor I had ever encountered.

As she walked toward the door, she stopped, turned toward me, and said, "I'm very competitive." I'm grateful that she is.

So what kind of doctors do you want, and how do you find them? First, you need a doctor who is an expert in your particular health problem. Friendly and charming is nice, but do you want your epitaph to be "He had a friendly and charming doctor"? Finding your expert is not hard. Start by googling your disease or medical issue, look for a treatment center or a foundation focused on helping people with this issue, and see who has received grants from the main federal agencies that fund scientific research, the National Institute of Health and the National Science Foundation. In a short time, you will have found the experts.

Then you must determine if this doctor sees patients or just does research. When you finally meet this doctor, give him or her a chemistry test: Is the chemistry between you and the doctor good? Does this doctor display empathy that reassures you that he or she will listen carefully to your concerns and give you the time you need to communicate the answers? Trust your judgment.

Now you are ready to find the best doctor for you.

One of the most telling ways to judge a doctor is by looking at how they communicate a scary diagnosis. I have received such diagnoses three times.

Doctors are taught to give bad news to patients by finding a quiet, private space and being direct, empathic, and understanding. They shouldn't rush, giving the patient time to process the news—or at least begin to process the news. It makes so much sense. I suppose it even works. But I have been given bad news—really bad news—three times, and the doctors were working from a totally different script.

The first time I received bad news was in 1995 when I was traveling from New York to Washington on the morning shuttle flight. As the president of the Hemophilia Association of New York, I had agreed to join a small group of doctors and hospital executives to lobby a group of government bureaucrats about how clotting factor—the lifesaving but incredibly expensive treatment for bleeding episodes—should be paid for those patients who were on Medicaid. I was sitting on a plane next to my hematologist at the time, an esteemed doctor nearing his retirement. He was by the window, and I was in the middle seat. This already made me uncomfortable because being squished into a middle seat on a crowded plane often makes me claustrophobic.

The doctor turned to me and said, "I have been meaning to tell you that you recently used clotting factor that was probably carrying mad cow disease."

Mad cow disease, or Creutzfeldt-Jakob disease, is a fatal degenerative brain disorder that typically starts with memory loss, progresses to poor coordination, and finally causes dementia. It is uniformly fatal, usually in less than a year. Did this doctor think I was going to process this news during the next twenty minutes of the flight, or just say "Thanks for the update" and shrug it off?

Actually, my first thought was "So this is where you decide to tell me this, you jackass?" My second thought was "I am dead." Over the next months, every time I had trouble recalling a name or remembering a phone number, I thought that this was the beginning of mad cow. After a year I hadn't developed any symptoms, so I was pretty sure I'd dodged this bullet. Now, nearly thirty years later, I *am* sure. Perhaps the doctor thought that sitting together on a flight would give us time to talk. I will give him the benefit of the doubt.

The second time I received bad news was in 2010 after I changed hospitals and met with one of their hepatologists. I told her my story and she scheduled me for an MRI to evaluate my liver.

A few days later, I was sitting in the waiting room of a city agency where some colleagues and I had a meeting to discuss my college's economic development program. My cellphone rang—it was the hepatologist from the hospital.

"I have the results from your MRI," she said.

"Thanks for calling," I said, unaware that this was like thanking the executioner before being hung. "You have advanced cirrhosis and liver cancer," she continued. "You should get yourself on a transplant list. Here is the name and number of the person here you should connect with."

I am sure the doctor felt there was urgency to give me this news so that I could start working to obtain a transplant. Of course, I could have traveled to the hospital in under an hour, met with the doctor, and received the news in a more humane way. So much for following medical training on delivering bad news.

I don't remember the rest of the call. Sitting in a waiting room with half dozen colleagues, I was numb. I followed them into a conference room and sat down. I think I even participated, rather like being on autopilot.

I knew that transplants are hard to obtain, require major surgery, and can leave you sick for the rest of what remains of your life. I thought my life was over.

Later that day I called my longtime trusted hematologist, Dr. Walsh, to inform him of the news. He put me in touch with Dr. Kim at the Mount Sinai Hospital transplant unit.

The third time I received bad news was after my evaluation for a transplant at Mount Sinai. Dr. Kim had already told me that I needed a transplant, but I had to know how quickly I needed it or whether some surgery to remove the tumor on my liver would buy me extra time.

Accompanied by my wife, I met a liver surgeon in a small consultation room. Congenial and well regarded by the other doctors, he told me that surgery was not a good option because I would likely bleed to death during the operation. Livers are like eight-pound sponges filled with arteries, veins, and blood. Surgery is always difficult but especially so on a cirrhotic liver. When a liver begins to deteriorate, it becomes cirrhotic, which makes this big sponge more difficult to have blood pass through. The body compensates by working extra hard to push blood entering the liver. This is called hepatic hypertension, and it makes it difficult for a liver to heal after surgery. I had hepatic hypertension.

I asked the surgeon how long I likely had if I didn't receive a transplant.

He responded, "Maybe a year." He was gracious, but said he had to leave. He had delivered his message. His work was done.

I couldn't move. My wife and I sat there after he left. After a few minutes, a nurse came in and said someone was waiting to use the room. I felt glued to the chair. "Please move to the waiting room," she told us.

How a doctor gives you bad news says so much about the type of person they are.

How a doctor communicates your scary diagnosis is a good predictor of how future interactions will go. If your doctor couldn't deliver your initial scary diagnosis in a humane, calm manner and give you the time to process it and ask questions, I wouldn't expect that future conversations will be any better. If you quickly see that the level of care and concern is not what you need, it is better to act sooner than later by looking for a new doctor.

Doctors are craftspeople.

Similar to a customer who calls a carpenter when a drawer on a cabinet won't close, patients show up when something hurts. Both doctors and craftspeople fix the problem as quickly as possible and they move on. But doctors should also be teachers. They should regard their role as sacred. They are asked to take important actions that impact the length and quality of their patients' lives. They are entrusted with confidential information that many patients share with no one else. And many patients look up to them as gods or near gods, as my parents did. Treating a patient as a ten-minute assignment followed by checking the appropriate boxes is a disgrace because of all the teaching opportunities missed.

When doctors engage with patients, they have the opportunity to teach them about their health and what they can do to maintain or improve their well-being. The doctor can assess the patient's knowledge and add to it in important ways by filling in the gaps. Moreover, a physician can provide motivation for the patient to improve their health regimen. Sadly, few doctors take the time to do this. If, after an interaction or two, you believe that a doctor is more interested in telling you what to do than in informing you about your situation and answering your questions, find another doctor.

Five Guidelines for Choosing the Right Doctor

1. **Choose a doctor who specializes in what you have.** If you have kidney cancer, find a specialist in kidney cancer—not just kidney disease or cancer but kidney cancer. The most experienced doctors work in specialized centers that focus on a specific disease.

2. **Find a doctor who is service-oriented.** There will come a time during your treatment when you want to reach your doctor quickly. Check with the staff and other longtime patients to confirm that this doctor responds to patients' needs without undue delay.

3. **Select a doctor who trained at a top hospital.** Doctors spend four years in medical school and then complete an internship for a year and a residency for two to three years. This is followed by a fellowship in their chosen specialty. Of course, where they attended medical school matters, but in my opinion, it is more important that they completed their post-graduate training in a hospital with a strong record for handling patients like valued

customers. Having been trained in such a system, doctors will bring those values and practices to their patients.

4. **Give your prospective doctor a chemistry test.** Well, not that kind of chemistry test. Give them the "personal chemistry" test to see if you feel comfortable with this person. For example, are you willing to share all the details of your health with your doctor? Do you feel that in addition to a professional relationship, there is a personal connection? Did the physician communicate relevant information and your diagnosis in a gentle way that allowed you time to ask as many questions as you wanted?

5. **Money, money, money.** Money shouldn't figure into your relationship with your doctor in the least. Most doctors who work in clinics or hospitals are salaried employees. Those in private or group practices share in the profits of the practice and are more like entrepreneurs. If you have the impression that the office looks fancy—think, expensive furniture—it might signal that the doctor values their decorator more than their patients. It might be a good time to move on.

Chapter 9

FAITH, HOPE, AND THE THREE STOOGES

I sat on the edge of the examination table in a claustrophobic treatment room alone. I had been told several weeks earlier that I would need a liver transplant and that without it, my life span was, at best, a year. But in this small room by myself, the reality sank in.

I was there for a checkup so I could be approved for a transplant. My hepatologist, Dr. Kim, had given me an exam that included palpating my liver to see if it changed size or density. She said nothing about the exam findings.

But then she said, "After you are transplanted, you will be on a regular schedule of bloodwork." Her assistant came in and asked her to take a call in another room.

Then it hit me: "After I am transplanted?" The words "after I am transplanted" went around and around in my head.

It was as if I had never been told I was very sick and needed a transplant. My mood fell, my blood pressure rose, my skin became clammy, and I felt trapped in this little prison cell.

Like everyone else, I was experiencing how a scary diagnosis takes control of your thoughts and emotions. You can't believe it. You can't understand it. You don't know if you can even make it through the day by yourself. Early thoughts will be of your family, your doctors, and any higher power you may feel connected to. These people will provide you with the emotional support, medical help, and confidence to fight this battle you are now joining. You will also rely upon your family, the healthcare system, and your community to find hope for a positive outcome. And you will find solace in *The Three Stooges Show*—or whatever brings you joy and laughter—so you continue to value life as you cope with the difficult days ahead.

The body and mind are, in many ways, tethered and yet independent of each other. You may become sad when you are sick or you may throw up defenses and feel just fine in a blissful state of denial. A positive disposition may keep you on a path of healthy habits, such as diet and exercise. A negative attitude may turn you into a noncompliant patient who refuses to take your medicine or keep doctors' appointments. People who feel supported by their families and friends may find the courage to tackle whatever illness has appeared. An isolated and lonely person may just want to curl up in a ball and let the disease have its way, the sooner the better.

As I sat in the treatment room waiting for Dr. Kim-Schluger to return, it was clear my mind was unconnected to my body and the reality that I had a very sick liver. Over the coming weeks before I was transplanted, my mind came to terms with the reality of my health and I developed my own strategies for coping. Having been sick with hemophilia and its impacts throughout my life, including many hospitalizations as a child, I had developed a resilience that I could now call on to help me once again.

This resilience had several components. While not religious, I have some manner of faith. When I found a doctor I had confidence in, as I did with Dr. Kim-Schluger, I had faith in her. When I experienced a hospital or clinic that I came to respect, I had faith in it. I have a wife who is unfailingly loving and supportive, so I have faith in her. My resilience included a positive attitude about life, which kept me hopeful and moving forward even during tough times. But alone in that treatment room I was challenged as never before and floundering too much to engage faith or hope or the Three Stooges. Yes.

Faith, hope, and the Three Stooges are tools that helped me build resilience. Perhaps it is surprising, but all have been studied and stand up to the rigors of scientific research.

Faith is complex. We most often associate it with religion and faith in God. In fact, the effects of faith on health as evidenced by participation in organized religion is associated with healthy behaviors such as lower rates of smoking, alcohol consumption, and drug use.

As Don Schepers discusses later in the book, faith without action is meaningless. Outcomes such as lower blood pressure and less severe heart disease are more common among people who practice religion. Immune function has also been found to be stronger in religious people. Recovery from medical procedures is faster, the ability to manage stress better, and the perception of pain lower in religious patients. Religious people even have longer life expectancies.

The first time I found my faith was as a five- or six-year-old tethered to an IV pole and hospital bed in the most profoundly lonely moment of my life. For that little boy, faith meant a connection to God, something that has waxed and waned for me in the decades since. But as I came to learn, faith has multiple dimensions. Of course, a belief and connection to a higher power is one. But as patients coping with a scary diagnosis, we can also place our faith in the doctors and other health professionals to whom we look for treatments and cures.

Health care almost always involves some type of treatment, and treatments vary greatly. Of course, pharmaceuticals, such as drugs, chemotherapy, or salves are the most common types of treatments. But many others—acupuncture, diet, rest, or stress reduction, for example—also exist. We put our faith in these as well. Although recently there is more controversy about how reliable a US Food and Drug Administration approval is, we generally have faith that drugs would not have been licensed without proof of their efficacy.

Studying anything as complex, variable, and hard to define as religion is difficult, and reaching unimpeachable results is nearly impossible. My conclusion is that people who have faith—regardless of what sort of faith—have a powerful tool to help them cope with a scary diagnosis.

People with positive attitudes are shown to cope better with illness than those with negative attitudes. The list of these positive outcomes reads just like the list for people of religious faith:

1. Stronger immune systems
2. Better cardiovascular health
3. Faster recoveries and healing
4. An enhanced ability to cope with mental stress and physical pain

People with positive attitudes live longer. I feel generally disposed to have a positive attitude. Where it comes from, I have no idea. Perhaps it's genetic. Perhaps I developed this ability through previous health crises when I emerged to again enjoy life.

But where do the Three Stooges fit in? Nothing creates a more positive attitude than laughing. I remember many times when I was hospitalized as a child, tethered to an IV pole and confined to bed, that I would watch *The Three Stooges Show* on the hospital television and laugh until tears ran down my cheeks. When I see these 1950s episodes today, I can fully understand that the core audience for the Three Stooges was boys between five and fifteen years old. Pratfalls, moronic behavior, and silliness are endlessly hysterical to them.

The scholar and author Norman Cousins contracted a crippling connective tissue disease when he was around fifty years old. When he was given little hope for a recovery, Cousins took matters into his own hands by treating himself with megadoses of vitamins and a regimen of laughter. He was past "the Three Stooges" phase of his development, so he moved on to the *Candid Camera* television show and comedy readings. In time, his symptoms began to ameliorate and then completely pass.

Cousins memorialized his journey in the book *Anatomy of an Illness as Perceived by the Patient*, which was later turned into a movie with the actor Ed Asner playing Cousins. In hindsight, his doctors questioned the diagnosis Cousins was given and argued that he might have recovered with or without laughter. Maybe so. But lots of laughter certainly reduced his pain, improved his mood, and gave him a feeling of control over his treatment.

I keep stressing one of the themes of the book is the importance of each patient's family and friends. Their support, the comfort and the connection to the real world that they provide, and their advocacy when needed are all central components of the healing process. Patients who have gone through long treatments and recoveries invariably thank their health-care providers and families in the same breath. When that faith in family and friends is proven unwarranted, the effects are devastating.

I had a good friend, I'll call him William, who had hemophilia and contracted HIV from a blood transfusion in the early 1980s. It was early in the epidemic, the cause of the disease was not certain, and there was no treatment. It did, however, soon become clear that the disease was transmitted sexually, as well as through blood transfusions and the shared needles of drug addicts.

William had been married to Barbara for about fifteen years, and it always seemed to me that his wife chose to look past William's physical limitations caused by decades of joint-destroying bleeds and chose to appreciate him as a brilliant, clever, and funny person. Barbara didn't involve herself in the frequent care that William required, such as visits to hospitals and the self-infusions of clotting factor that William administered himself at home.

But when William showed signs of HIV, it was too much for Barbara. When William returned from work one day, Barbara and all her things were gone. William was understandably shattered as the faith and trust he had placed in his wife was revealed as misplaced.

I had witnessed William's resilience over the years. He was always in pain from his damaged joints and struggled to walk with a cane, but he remained funny and hopeful. It took a couple of years for William to recover from Barbara's abandoning him, but he *did* recover and went on to have the happiest, most secure relationship of his life with a sonographer whom he met at the hospital.

I previously introduced you to Don Schepers, a colleague and friend of mine who has Parkinson's. He spent twenty-five years as a Catholic priest before concluding that he was feeling increasingly out of place and decided to leave the priesthood and pursue a PhD in organizational behavior and an academic career as a professor and scholar. Around this time Don married a religious sister, Jeanne.

I asked Don about how faith informed his coping with his illness. I couldn't say it better than he did:

> The questions you pose have so many different answers, depending on one's view of God. For instance, I'm not one to ask "Why me?" sorts of questions, as if God meted out this as some sort of test or punishment. I can't answer for those people.
>
> I experience my life as a bifurcated existence: part logical positivist, part faithful Catholic. The scientist in me demands the perspective of the logical positivist: if it can't be proven, it doesn't exist. This works fine for the real world, and the operations of science. Deduction, induction, and all the methods of evidence gathering and reasoning work well in this venue.
>
> How, then, do I approach the question of God? Evidence and reason are clearly not the coin of the realm. And however one approaches the scriptures (Jewish, Christian, Muslim, or any permutation thereof), the simple fact is that they are religious lore—stories meant

to imbue faith—not record historical events. There may be some history, but the primary intended effect is the fostering of faith, both at the individual and communal levels.

How to Marshal the Three Powerful Forces of Faith, Hope, and the Three Stooges

Faith. If you are a religious person and have clergy with whom you feel comfortable, you might engage in a discussion of what your faith says about scary diagnoses and coping with illness. As Don eloquently noted, this might be a good time to strengthen your connection to your community of faith.

Hope. You need to make getting your attitude pointed in the right—that is, positive—direction a priority. This can be accomplished by connecting with people who have had your diagnosis and recovered or by looking at the statistics on health outcomes for people in your situation. Even if your prognosis is poor, you can still have hope that you will receive loving and supportive care up until your death. You can also button up any uncompleted personal or family business, such as reconnecting with friends, relatives, and business partners from whom you have become estranged. Helping family and loved ones accept a poor prognosis and play a supportive role in achieving a "good death" for the patient is something to expect from the medical staff.

The Three Stooges. Like Norman Cousins, find ways to laugh and experience joy. Perhaps it will improve the likelihood of a good health outcome. But even if it doesn't, experiencing as much joy, happiness, and love as possible is a wonderful thing.

Chapter 10

TO SHARE OR NOT TO SHARE

I was a young child when my parents made the decision to keep my hemophilia a secret. This had many negative repercussions. It created a bifurcated world for me: those who knew I had hemophilia and those who didn't. Worse than that, it signaled to me that hemophilia was something that I should be ashamed of and could be used against me.

But there was one positive result of this decision: keeping me mainstreamed in school and out of the "special needs" program. In the 1950s, children with health issues and special needs were lumped together and segregated in their own classes, with programs more focused on keeping them physically safe than intellectually challenged. These students' academic goals were sacrificed. I see now that I was early proof of the value of mainstreaming students with physical disabilities to the greatest extent possible.

While we have a long way to go, the 1950s attitudes about illness have evolved into greater emphasis on ensuring that people with health challenges—whether they be physical or mental disabilities—are not shunted aside.

This is generally called mainstreaming, and it's a good thing. People with physical disabilities and health challenges are capable of high-level functioning in many ways, and the more the general population sees this, the better off everyone will be.

A corollary of this is that people with disabilities feel less shame and embarrassment than they might have decades ago, and the general population is less judgmental of them

There may be less of a choice in telling others when a scary diagnosis is followed by an apparent disability because of treatment—such as losing one's hair because of chemotherapy or walking with crutches because of leg surgery.

But what about when a diagnosis or its treatment does not lead to any obvious effects? Should you tell people? And whom should you tell?

After receiving a scary diagnosis, you face the decision of whom to tell. Telling some people may be incredibly useful, while telling others won't benefit you. So how do you decide?

The writer Nora Ephron was diagnosed with leukemia and managed the difficult chemotherapy treatments while telling only a handful of people about her health crisis. Of course, writers often lead isolated lives. If you desire to keep your diagnosis a secret, ask yourself if that's even a realistic option given your day-to-day life.

If you own a retail store, work in a law office, or are a soccer coach, maintaining any such secrecy would be tough. Deciding whom you will tell requires planning.

- Is your illness a secret?
- If so, who can be trusted to keep your secret?
- How will you communicate with others during the period of being sick, being treated, and missing work?

Some people are incredibly open about their medical issues, both past and present. At a friend's birthday party, a woman I'd never met before introduced herself to me as a cancer survivor. I had been so thoroughly trained by my parents over the course of a lifetime to keep my hemophilia secret that her openness struck me as a type of exhibitionism. But if such openness is a constructive coping mechanism that makes you feel more comfortable in your sick-person skin, go for it!

Growing up, I carefully rationed the truth about my health status. I kept a mental record of who knew and who didn't know. The circle of those who knew gradually grew over the years, but secrets also flourished.

I hid my chronic hepatitis and being at risk for HIV, especially during the years when AIDS was feared but not understood. I rationed the truth about my need for a liver transplant, then hid it when I received a new liver.

I didn't want people asking me about where I was on the list to be matched to a liver or what my alternatives might be, since there were none.

I didn't want people treating me like a fragile butterfly or making me a topic of conversation and gossip.

Because I worked in a college and received my transplant in July, my work schedule allowed me to be away for three weeks with no one the wiser. When I returned at the beginning of the fall semester, people noticed I was thinner, which was not a bad thing. I toyed with the idea of telling people I went to a spa for three weeks. In the end, I let them imagine the improbable idea that I had been on a diet.

As I stated earlier, many people coping with illness divide the world in two: those who know about and can even share in your experience, and those who can't.

There may be people who you *don't* want to bring into this highly personal and intimate part of your life.

I can't understate the importance of having a community of your peers and friends to help you cope with illness.

Six Guidelines for Sharing Your Health Information

1. **Share if you must.** If you have no choice because your condition causes hair loss or obvious physical disability, it may be difficult to remain silent, and you have to say something. You may choose to tell the whole detailed story or you may tell a shortened and minimized version: "It looks worse than it is. The doctors are optimistic, and I should be 100 percent in a few months." If people probe for more, it's okay to say, "I don't feel comfortable going through all the details, but thank you for your concern."

2. **Tell your team.** As I discussed earlier, when this adventure started, you built a team to support you. This might include family, friends, and colleagues. The more they know and the closer they are to the truth of your scary diagnosis, the more supportive and helpful they can be.

3. **Be selective at work.** If your condition or its treatment doesn't compromise your job performance, it's none of their business. If you need accommodations at work, it is probably best to first discuss it with the staff in Human Resources because they know (or should know) the law.

4. **Become familiar with family and medical leave laws.** Federal Family and Medical Leave Act (FMLA) grants twelve weeks of unpaid leave for people coping with serious medical issues for yourself or a family member. It only applies to organizations with fifty or more

employees. Also, about a dozen states have passed their own FMLA laws, which provide twelve weeks of paid leave in such cases. If you must access this system, learn as much about it as possible as soon as possible.

5. **Maintain your boundaries.** As much as you need to share your medical information with your doctors and nurses, you should always regard it as your personal and private information. Unless there is some specific benefit to sharing your health information, keep it private.

6. **Never forget that you are not your diagnosis.** There are times when your diagnosis will overwhelm and preoccupy you, but other aspects of your life—family, work, interests, and friends—should remain important. Maintaining your focus on positive parts of your life will help remind you that you are so much more than just a scary diagnosis.

Chapter 11

MANAGING THE HOSPITAL EXPERIENCE

People sometimes confuse hospitals with hotels. They think there's a TripAdvisor category for hospitals that ranks them by the food, the comfiness of the beds, the friendliness of the staff, the enthusiasm of the tanning concierge, and the price of parking, among other perks.

Let's be clear: your goals when checking out these institutions should be quite different. In a hotel, you want to depart well rested, relaxed, and with a few new friends. As a hospital patient, your goal is to avoid permanently "checking out." Irrelevant to this goal is whether the curtains on the windows meet your aesthetic standards, the food is good, the thread count of the sheets is in the double—if not triple—digits, and if the wait for the elevator is annoyingly long.

In other words, get over it! You have bigger fish to fry.

You are going to a hospital to undergo tests and receive a diagnosis, to have surgery, or to undergo treatments and supportive care while your body struggles with a health crisis. You really have no choice. There is no other place in the world with the equipment and expertise to achieve these results. So let go of your desire for a good night's sleep, yummy food, and high-thread-count sheets. Focus on achieving your health goals and exiting through the lobby, not the morgue.

As I noted earlier, about two-thirds of US hospitals are nonprofits (American Hospital Association Annual Reports). About a quarter of hospitals are profit-making, and the balance—about 19 percent—are public or government owned. But just because a hospital is organized as a nonprofit doesn't mean they want to lose money. Regardless of their profit-making or nonprofit status, they all work incredibly hard not only to break even but to do even better.

Generally hospitals do better financially when they treat patients with private insurance, perform lots of surgeries and procedures, and provide highly specialized care. This is because they can charge more for these services.

The Cleveland Clinic, where I had my liver transplant, is a nonprofit, but it is highly prosperous. It is one of the top heart treatment hospitals in the world, which means it performs thousands of successful heart surgeries. It attracts wealthy patients from all over the globe who either have private insurance or bulging wallets in need of surgical reduction. The bill for my liver transplant was $450,000, although in all likelihood the Cleveland Clinic collected less than that from my private insurer. It cost me only a twenty-five-dollar co-pay, a three-week stay in a budget motel on the hospital's campus, meals in local restaurants, and a plane ticket home.

To bolster their bottom lines, both private and nonprofit hospitals have focused on certain money-making procedures.

These include maternity and ultra-premier services such as private rooms and chef-prepared food for wealthy patients who can pay and pay and pay. Hospitals compete for maternity patients by offering private rooms, an extra bed for dad, luxury surroundings, high-thread-count sheets, and an in-room champagne post-delivery dinner for the new parents. Very nice.

But the most important issue is that mother and baby leave the hospital healthy. There is a line between good care in comfortable surroundings and high-thread-count sheets. The reality is that when the baby is ready to emerge, the last thing on the mother's mind is luxurious amenities.

As noted above, indulging the ultra-rich is another money-maker for hospitals. There is a population of sheiks, oligarchs, and Silicon Valley billionaires who are willing to pay for the privilege to have a four-star chef cook their favorite foods as they recover from hemorrhoid surgery or to listen to Mozart in their private room while the doctor checks their scar following bariatric surgery. The question is whether these folks actually receive better care in the bargain. It varies by hospital, but I doubt it.

The best care is provided when experienced and expert staff is constantly available and checking on the patient. The best care is provided on floors serving multiple patients with similar conditions and staff who are familiar with their needs. I would rather be near a highly experienced nurse than a four-star chef when I am in the hospital.

Never forget that when you are in the hospital, you are not just a patient; you are a customer. The hospital is hoping to receive more from your insurance company than they spend on your care. In other words, the hospital sees you as its own little profit center. When the doctor tells you that you can go home following your gall bladder removal surgery, they may be pressured because your insurance company pays the hospital a fixed amount for this surgery and follow-up care. Taking a day off your hospital stay reduces their cost of taking care of you without reducing incoming revenue from another insurance company.

But what if the hospital wants to send you home and you don't feel ready?

Perhaps you don't feel steady on your feet, or the person who was going to provide home care has canceled, or you're just too worried to leave the hospital. In this argument—if that's what it becomes—you should expect that your doctor will be your advocate with the hospital or insurance company. Hospitals provide patient advocates to help with this process as well. But you may have to seek out such assistance.

Even with the constant activity of staff running up and down the halls, patients being moved in wheelchairs and on gurneys or shuffling along with their IV poles in tow, there can be tremendous loneliness. I find isolation the greatest negative of being in a hospital. If your condition gives you the mobility to sit in a lounge area, then make that part of your routine.

Patients are cut off from their friends and families. They're also removed from all the activities they love and that provide them comfort, including their pets and their favorite foods, so their minds wander to their pain and fear.

Five Guidelines for Maintaining Sanity in the Hospital

1. **Create distractions.** Reading, knitting, watching every Academy Award–nominated film on your iPad, and, of course, having visitors.

2. **Sleep, then sleep some more.** Besides sleep being restorative, it helps the time pass. If you can't sleep, ask for pharmaceutical help.

3. **Exercise by walking the halls,** even it means you are pushing your IV pole and your butt is hanging out because the hospital gowns are designed for those most proud of their posteriors. Just ask for a second gown and wear it backward.

4. **Block out noise.** Hospitals are noisy places, and much of the noise—such as staff running through the halls to the latest emergency or the alarms on the IV drip machines telling the staff to replenish the fluid—is unsettling. Bring noise-canceling earbuds or headphones, listen to your favorite music, and tune out the hospital.

5. **Have your visitors sit with you for as much time as you both can tolerate.** Perhaps you can play cards or discuss a recent family wedding. In my experience, just sitting in the company of someone you love will do more to relax you than anything else.

"Will I ever get better? How long until this pain recedes?" Throughout my hospitalizations as a child and an adult, I came to the conclusion that any distraction was better than none. The most readily available distraction in a hospital is a roommate. People who prefer private rooms in hospitals may be confusing hospitals with hotels.

Many people are afraid of sharing a room in a hospital. We are taught to believe that a private room in an office, a hotel, or a sleeper on a train is always better—it's more expensive but you can expect a good night's sleep.

Sorry, Charlie. In a hospital, you should not expect to have a good night's sleep. Your blood pressure and other vital signs will be taken every few hours. You may be awakened to take them. If you are on an IV drip, when the fluids run low, the regulator machine will beep like a frustrated cab driver stuck behind a slow-moving garbage truck. In my opinion, you might as well have some company or even some entertainment, which may be provided by a roommate.

But there is another reason to share a room. You are in the hospital because you need medical attention you can't receive anywhere else.

Being in a room with another patient guarantees that you will be seen by more nurses, aides, and doctors.

A roommate might hear you if you need help. In theory, the nurses' station responds to the buzzer you are given precisely for the purpose of summoning help or at least requesting help. If you are asking for more water, to have your bed adjusted, or to pick up the pillow that fell on the floor, you will likely wait a long time. But if there is a nurse at the next bed helping your roommate, you can ask for anything and receive an immediate response. Even for more serious matters, such as uneven breathing while you are sleeping, a nurse caring for your roommate is more likely to take notice and take action.

Most roommates are in similar situations. Perhaps both of you had joint replacements or are undergoing chemotherapy. This gives you a topic to discuss, perhaps learn from each other and even bond. But regardless of whether your roommate and you talk to each other, the presence of a roommate creates distraction and even engagement. Of course, it doesn't always work out that way.

Watching or hearing a half dozen medical personnel work feverishly to revive your roommate (the nurses will pull the curtain to give some weak semblance of privacy) will not lift your spirits. Smelling someone use a bedpan, listening to your roommate's calls begging for visitors, or hearing groans and farts will make you wish for a private room. But that has not been my main experience of hospital roommates.

A few months before I had my liver transplant, I had an upper endoscopy, a test in which a tube with a camera on the end was snaked down my esophagus and into my stomach. I was, of course, under anesthesia. During the process, the tube tore a varicose vein in my esophagus and it started to bleed. For patients with advanced liver disease, such as cirrhosis, the development of varicose veins in the esophagus is common because the high blood pressure in the liver puts extra strain on these veins; they weaken and are easily broken.

The doctor doing the endoscopy had not encountered a hemophilia patient before and panicked. The doctor was told by the hematologist on call to administer clotting factor to me and to calm herself down. She did this and the bleeding stopped, but I was admitted to the hospital to make sure this wasn't going to reoccur. I was put in a room on an internal medicine floor of patients with various ailments. I had a roommate. I was relieved—at least initially.

My roommate was an elderly man who was unconscious and connected to at least a half dozen tubes. These tubes ended in plastic bags arrayed on the floor beneath his bed in a Jackson Pollock–like display of colors: brown, green, yellow, and clear. Above his bed, several IV bags delivered various medications directly into his veins. So I assumed I would have a quiet roommate.

My roommate had four relatives who stayed by his side, even refusing to leave when visiting hours had ended. They all spoke Russian, except whenever the nurse asked them something and they explained that the patient only spoke Russian. This meant, they said, they had to stay by his side to translate.

First of all, this poor fellow wasn't saying anything in any language. He was comatose. Second, the hospital employs translators. Nonetheless, the relatives weren't leaving. When they got hungry, they dug into several shopping bags of food, mostly fragrant smoked meats. When they became sleepy, they nodded off and snored with enthusiasm. When they became bored, they turned on the television to the local cable news channel—in English—that repeated the same stories several times per hour.

Bad enough? No. Earlier that day, Dr. Jack Kevorkian had died. Kevorkian, known by the moniker Dr. Death, believed in assisted suicide for terminally ill patients. Now my roommate's TV was set on a channel that broadcast Dr. Kevorkian's obituary several times an hour.

I couldn't sleep because of my roommate's relatives. Also, I had hiccups from the endoscopy. The hiccups wouldn't quit. So there I sat at the edge of my bed, looking at a man likely at death's door, listening to his family talk and snore, smelling their aromatic but unappetizing food, and hearing the news of Dr. Kevorkian's death over and over and over—and hiccupping. It was not a good night.

But guess what? As annoying as these family members were, it was better to witness their show than to be isolated in a private room.

A Few Tools to Cope with Hospital Roommates and Their Guests

1. **It is best to connect with your roommate.** You may be able to help each other such as calling for help to changing the television channel.
2. **Don't pry.** You will be curious about what brought your roommate to this situation in his or her life. While you

may be willing to share your story, not everyone is. If you volunteer your story, most roommates will respond in kind.

3. **You are not the entertainment for visitors.** Most visitors really don't want to be there. Hospitals make many people anxious and visiting a sick relative or friend brings up fears. As a distraction your roommate's visitors may turn to you to tell your story and chat with them. I always resented this. If you are like me, tell them you need to rest.

Chapter 12

COPING WITH BIG, BAD BUREAUCRACIES

Let's try to understand these monsters that make up the health-care system bureaucracy by eliminating a few misconceptions you may have. First, the health-care system doesn't exist or operate primarily for your benefit. The health-care system mostly comprises gargantuan capitalistic organizations whose primary goals include making profits, paying executives huge salaries, growing their organizations even bigger, and achieving high rankings so they can attract more patients and charge even higher prices. In the process of working toward these goals, they also cure diseases, apply the latest in technology and science, and often treat their patients with respect and care. Play your cards right and you can be one of those lucky patients.

My high school Latin teacher taught me that the Latin word *patiens* means "one who suffers" and is the origin of the English word *patient*. Draw your own conclusions. You don't want to be one for whom the Latin word is most apt. It is my purpose in this chapter to present the reality of the health-care system to you so that you can understand and maneuver through the system, get the most benefit, and suffer the least in the process.

I realize that I have already misspoken. Yes, I would like you to understand the system, but frankly it just isn't possible. No one does. Maneuvering through the complexities of health insurance can be difficult and fraught with danger for anyone. Even someone who has a good job, health insurance, money in the bank, and experience managing financial and health-care issues can be flummoxed. Consider the three-year saga of my friend Mark Gibbel.

Mark was the vice president of development for the New School for Social Research in New York. "Development," also known as fundraising, is a very important effort for every nonprofit organization, including universities like the New School. During Mark's employment there, the New School provided health insurance, initially, through Aetna. I'll call this Plan #1. Then the university changed plans to UnitedHealthcare in a cost-saving move. I'll call this Plan #2.

Changing health insurance is a major pain for all the policyholders. It requires updating the doctors, hospitals, and clinics you use, as well as closing out the remaining bills with your previous insurer. Often it requires the policyholder to change doctors because not every doctor accepts every plan. But Mark was certainly capable of managing these tasks, if he could make the time to do so. Soon after the UnitedHealthcare plan took effect, Mark decided to retire. If he had been sixty-five years old or older, he would have been eligible for Medicare, the federal insurance plan. Since he wasn't yet sixty-five, he had to choose COBRA coverage, which I'll call Plan #3. He stayed on COBRA for eighteen punishing months.

A cobra is a snake that kills its prey by injecting it with venom through its fangs. The venom stops the prey's heart from beating and its lungs from breathing. COBRA insurance overwhelms its policyholders with insane rules and huge amounts of paperwork until it makes their heads explode. COBRA is an acronym for Consolidated Omnibus Budget Reconciliation Act, which was passed by Congress in 1985 and signed by President Ronald Reagan in 1986. On January 20, 1981, when he was inaugurated as president, Reagan said, "Government is not the solution to our problem; government *is* the problem." Nothing Reagan ever did proved this truer than creating the COBRA health insurance system.

COBRA is meant to provide a continuity of health insurance for those who leave their jobs or are fired. It gives the former employee coverage but entirely at their own expense and not necessarily through the same insurer who provided their coverage while they were employed. Mark was offered COBRA from UnitedHealthcare, his Plan #3. The price was $3,250 per month for his family. Then he developed kidney stones.

Kidney stones are recognized as one of the most painful ailments a person can endure. The pain comes and goes, but when a person passes a stone through the narrow urinary tract, the pain is comparable to childbirth. Mark's urologist did not accept UnitedHealthcare, but both the doctor and the hospital gave Mark a 20 percent discount on their usual charges, which left Mark with a bill of $12,000. Insurance paid nothing. One year of COBRA saw the removal of his kidney stones from his urinary tract and the extraction of $51,000 from his bank account for the insurance policy, the doctor's bill, and the hospital's charges. So, Mark decided to try Obamacare.

The Affordable Care Act, nicknamed Obamacare, went into effect in 2014 and was intended to provide health insurance to any individual under sixty-five (after which they can receive

Medicare) without regard to preexisting conditions. Certain standards were set, such as providing preventative care, vaccines, and screening for common diseases. Mark looked up the price of an Obamacare policy in New York State and saw that it was $2,400 per month. It was expensive, but it was about $850 per month less than he was paying for COBRA. This was Plan #4, and he remained on Obamacare for a year.

After this year, Mark was rejected for an Obamacare renewal because he was not working and he had no income. The Obamacare representative told Mark he needed to go on Medicaid, which covers people living in poverty. I will call this Plan #5. None of his health-care providers accepted Medicaid, so Mark changed to another Medicaid plan. This became Plan #6. Mark was actually pleased with the health care he received under Medicaid. The customer service was excellent, well above the (dis)service he had received from Aetna or UnitedHealthcare.

Then Mark turned sixty-five and had to change to Medicare, which I'll call Plan #7.

Seven insurance plans in three years, out-of-pocket expenses well over $50,000, long delays in receiving treatment, and then the COVID-19 pandemic hit. Hospitals told him not to show up. He would not be allowed into the building because every bed was taken with COVID-19 patients who were accepted regardless of whether they had insurance. Meanwhile, Mark was again suffering attacks of kidney stone pain. Finally, the pandemic receded and Mark was able to have his current crop of kidney stones removed and start a treatment regimen that would prevent any more from developing.

Most developed countries in the world have single-payer insurance in which one organization, generally a quasi-governmental agency, provides health care to everyone—employed or unemployed—as a basic human right. Mark's trek through seven expensive and inadequate insurance policies in three years is a good argument for this system.

The health-care system is complex beyond any human capacity for comprehension. I don't think that if Siri, Alexa, Watson, ChatGPT, and six chess grandmasters collaborated, they could read your insurance guidebook and tell you the co-pay for having your bunions removed. The largest companies in the health-care system employ thousands of lawyers, and a good portion of their time is spent arguing over what the laws that Congress and fifty state legislatures have enacted actually mean and if they should pay your medical bills.

Anyway, let's dive in. Perhaps I have scared you too much. Yes, it is impossible to understand the health-care system fully, but it is possible for you to understand enough about the basics to make good decisions on where to go for your care and how to manage the system to obtain the best care possible. Let's get started by identifying the main monsters, what they do, and how a patient can manage them.

Private versus Nonprofit versus Public

A few fundamental distinctions will greatly help you grasp both the insurance and health-care system.

Private Companies

Virtually all pharmaceutical companies are privately owned for-profit private companies. They are owned by their shareholders, and generally issue and trade their shares in the stock markets such as the New York Stock Exchange or the NASDAQ exchange. They pay taxes, raise capital to grow by issuing bonds or more stock, and can merge with one another or sell off parts of their companies as their management and shareholders wish. They are maniacally driven to increase their profits, generally measured by earnings per share, which will then lead their stock prices.

Nonprofit Organizations

St. Jude, Mayo Clinic, Kaiser Permanente, and others have chosen to avoid the business status and accept the benefits of being nonprofits. A nonprofit designation is really a tax status, designated as a 501(c)3, the IRS tax code section that governs them.

Unlike businesses that report primarily to their shareholders, nonprofits don't pay taxes, can accept donations that are tax-deductible to the donors, and report to their state charity bureaus. It is a common misconception to assume that an organization with a nonprofit designation is run strictly for the public good. Perhaps, but probably not. Nonprofit organizations have to balance their books just as profit-making businesses do. Nonprofits don't make profits but they do create surpluses, which are effectively the same. I have worked with some of the largest nonprofit hospital groups in the US and know that their leaders work just as hard to create financial surpluses as any private business CEO works to make a profit. Surpluses can be used to improve services, allow them to expand facilities, and—most importantly—raise the salaries of their executives.

Public Organizations

Public organizations are divisions of a government. Medicare, Medicaid, Social Security, Obamacare, and the Veterans Administration are all examples of huge public health-care–related organizations. They exist to provide insurance to specific groups of people defined by public service, age, income, and health status. They are not necessarily free. Some are paid for by withholdings from salary checks such as Social Security. Medicare has a basic plan but also offers the option to pay more for fuller coverage. Obamacare has fees, but they are generally low because they are subsidized by the federal government.

Employers and unions can also play major roles in health care by providing insurance that is generally negotiated through large insurance companies and by negotiating with health-care providers for lower prices.

Insurance

If you are like most people, as soon as you hear the word *insurance*, your brain freezes. My goal is to unfreeze your brain enough to understand what the health-care insurance system is, how this vicious monster came to be, and how you can tame it. I believe that when you see the context in which the system operates and have some guidelines for your interaction with it, your anxiety will recede.

Insurance operates with a simple business model. We all pay in, and when individuals need money, they can take it out. This could be fire insurance, car insurance, flood insurance, or life insurance. The entity that runs the pool could be a private company, a nonprofit organization, or a government agency. Of course, this entity needs to at least break even, and its business model is simple. It takes in money from premiums and earns money by investing the funds it holds before it pays claims. Money goes out by paying claims and the administrative costs of managing the process. Carefully and thoughtfully done, it is a good business. But if the company sells flood insurance in an area before a huge storm, or sells life insurance before a pandemic, the outflows may exceed the inflows and the company can go bankrupt.

In today's world, insurance companies rarely go bankrupt because government regulators check that they are not taking untoward risks. Plus insurance companies themselves hold insurance from reinsurance companies to reimburse them for unexpected losses. But this doesn't make them generous or even reasonable. Every dollar they save by *not* paying for your medical costs or the costs of rebuilding your home after a fire is profit for them. Some insurance companies play this game with a brutality that even the ruthless Soviet dictator Joseph Stalin would envy.

I have never been able to wrap my head around the fact that the wealthiest nation in the history of the world cannot provide health care to all of its citizens. According to the Census Bureau 26 million Americans or 7.9 percent of the population have no health insurance. Many more have inadequate coverage, and everyone with insurance realizes that it is devilishly and infuriatingly complex.

The health insurance business is a combination of Whac-a-Mole, pinball, and three-level chess. It will infuriate you, impoverish you, and make you sick to your stomach. It is difficult enough to deal with when you are feeling perfectly well and just earned a joint law degree and PhD in econometrics. But if you never got past twelfth-grade math, struggle with English, are trying to hold down two jobs, and are ill, you are simply overmatched when an insurance giant who doesn't care if you live or die decides it wants you to pay for your own care, even if that forces you into financial ruin.

But imagine this: The president of the United States takes the podium in Congress to urge the adoption of a national health insurance program for every American. Insurance would cover all medical costs but also reimburse participants for lost wages. In this plan, doctors' bills and prescription drugs would be fully covered. You actually don't need to imagine this because on November 19, 1945, President Harry Truman addressed Congress with precisely this message.

While President Truman was promoting this proposal, the United States was guiding the rebuilding of the Axis powers in the aftermath of World War II. These efforts included creating democratic governments, Western-type judicial systems, and universal health care—which these countries all have today. In fact, the United States is the only developed country in the world without universal health care.

What we have built instead of a unified, efficient, and universal insurance system is a highly fractured jigsaw puzzle with at least a dozen types of insurance, thousands of different policies, and an administrative superstructure comprising one of the largest elements of health-care cost. In fact, about a quarter of all health-care expenditures support this administrative bloat, which includes nearly a quarter of a million people whose jobs are to code medical records for payment from insurers. How much better would health care be if these people were nurses?

Private insurance companies such as Aetna and Cigna focus on selling insurance coverage to large employers. This is a smart business strategy because people who work are generally healthy, so the costs to provide their care are lower than average.

Public insurance programs, such as Medicare and Medicaid, are focused on specific groups. Medicare is provided to people over sixty-five who no longer have private insurance through their work. Medicaid is for poor groups, but eligibility requirements vary by state.

Employment-related insurance is generally subcontracted to large private insurers such as Blue Cross Blue Shield, but the human resource departments of companies serve as gateways to the policies and issues related to coverage.

How Insurance Pays for Your Health Care

Insurance companies create schedules of payments to health-care providers who are willing to accept their insurance. With the largest institutions, insurance companies will negotiate individual reimbursement schedules. On the other side of the equation, the insurance company will offer policies to employers that require the employer and the employees to pay part of the premiums and the employee to pay some direct share of the health-care services they receive. This is called the co-pay.

Veterans Administration Health-Care System

The federal government spends over $300 billion on health-care services for veterans. Veterans pay fees in addition to that federal contribution. The cost structure for veterans receiving care from the US Department of Veterans Affairs (VA) can vary depending on several factors, such as their eligibility status, service-connected disabilities, income level, and priority groups based on eight factors including degree of disability, Medicaid status, and income.

Many veterans, particularly those with service-connected disabilities or those who meet low-income thresholds, qualify for free or low-cost health-care services through the VA. However, some veterans may have co-pays for certain types of care, depending on their income and the specific services received. Reservists are generally not entitled to health-care benefits unless they were injured in the line of duty.

The VA offers a comprehensive benefits package, including affordable health insurance options through the Veterans Health Administration (VHA) for veterans who do not meet the eligibility criteria for free health care. These insurance options allow veterans to access care outside the VA system and may require them to pay premiums and co-pays based on their income and health coverage plan.

Overall, the VA health-care system strives to provide accessible and affordable health-care services to veterans. The cost to veterans can vary depending on factors such as eligibility, income, and the specific services received, but the goal is to ensure that veterans receive the care they need without facing excessive financial burdens.

The Hospitals

There are over 5,570 hospitals in the US: 2,978 are organized as nonprofits, 1,150 are government owned and run, and 1,235 are for-profits (American Hospital Association Annual Report 2023). As I pointed out earlier, just because a hospital is organized as a nonprofit doesn't mean it can tolerate losses.

Public hospitals trace their origins to the "poor houses" of the eighteenth century that provided care to those without insurance or their own resources. While that perception may persist somewhat today, contemporary public hospitals are well staffed and equipped, and they accept insurance. However, because of their locations in poorer communities, they may have fewer patients with insurance and therefore need significant government subsidies.

Regardless of their organizational structure, all hospitals make more money when they treat patients with private insurance, because private insurance generally has higher reimbursement rates than Medicare and Medicaid. They also make more money when their care focuses on complex surgeries and procedures such as those performed by cardiology, oncology, and obstetrics departments—for example, heart bypass surgeries, cancer surgeries and treatments, and obstetrics. Think about it—aren't these the most common ways hospitals advertise themselves?

You need to consider the type of hospital you are thinking of using, the types of care they focus on, and their reputation.

The Pharmaceutical Companies

The pharmaceutical industry is incredibly profitable. A 2020 study published in the Journal of the American Medical Association (see references at end of book) reported that pharmaceutical companies over the ten years were twice as profitable as the rest of the publicly traded companies. In 2021, Pfizer had $42 billion in revenue and $16 billion in profits. Johnson & Johnson had $45 billion in revenue and earned $14 billion in profits. Merck garnered $51 billion in revenue and a pathetic $12 billion in profits.

What explains these huge profits? Congress. Federal law has given protections and support to pharmaceutical companies that other businesses can only envy. First, the research that leads to new drugs is largely funded by the federal government through the National Science Foundation and the National Institutes of Health. Private foundations, such as large health charities, also fund research to find treatments and cures for the diseases they focus on. Historically this government and private funding has provided more than half of the money spent on drug research, and sales of pharmaceuticals keep soaring. The pharmaceutical companies focus their spending on commercializing the outcomes of the basic research that the government and foundations have underwritten. Commercialization includes designing, manufacturing, packaging, and marketing their drugs.

Second, drugs are patent protected for twenty years, beginning when the patent application is filed. Because new drugs require a lengthy and expensive period of testing prior to receiving FDA approval before the company can sell the drug, the effective period of patent protection is closer to ten years. This still provides each company with ten years to sell the drug without any direct competition. Third, Congress enables drug companies to fix the price of their drugs. Only recently has Congress allowed Medicare, which purchases over $112 billion in drugs annually, to negotiate with the manufacturers to obtain lower, more reasonable prices.

What other business has the government underwrite their research development, grant them a monopoly to sell what comes from that research, and then allows them to fix the prices of their products?

Now you know why pharmaceutical companies are so profitable.

When the patent expires, other companies can produce the same drug and sell it as a generic. Without the upfront research and development costs already covered by the originating company and its funding sources, and absent the need for extensive testing and huge spending on marketing, generic drug manufacturers can undercut the price of the name brand. In addition, several generic drug manufacturers are likely competing with one another, contributing pressure to cut prices. Some people are skittish about purchasing generics, but there is no evidence generic drugs are less effective than the original brand name. Given the choice, especially if you spend your money on drugs, look for the generics and have your doctor prescribe them.

Distribution Companies

Another reason that drugs are so expensive is that distribution is handled by a small group of very large companies, including McKesson, AmerisourceBergen, Express Scripts, and a few others. Similarly, the retail pharmacy industry is dominated by just a few giants: CVS, Rite Aid, and Walgreens.

Because there are so few of these companies, they don't have much competition. This industry is an example of what economists call "stickiness," because once your prescription is with one company, it is difficult for you to change to another pharmacy and it is easy for them to raise prices. Other industries that benefit from this stickiness are cable TV and telephone companies. All of them end up having a great deal of control over their prices because of a lack of competition and the complex logistics involved for a consumer to switch companies.

We have recently seen some new entrants into the pharmaceutical distribution business such as Amazon and Mark Cuban Cost Plus Drugs. Time will tell if they will be able to attract enough customers to thrive or even survive.

Doctors

When I was a sick child, my parents would call a doctor who would come to the house carrying a black leather bag with a stethoscope, other small tools, and a small pharmacy. My parents paid him in cash. Those days are gone. Today, the vast majority of doctors are employed by hospitals or clinics.

According the American Medical Association, the share of physicians working in private practices, or those wholly-owned by physicians, fell by 13 percent between 2012 and 2022 — from 60.1 to 46.7 percent. The implication for patients is troublesome. A doctor in private practice is likely to remain in private practice for most of their careers. A doctor employed by a large medical institution is more likely to move around within their institution and less likely to maintain a steady group of patients in their practice. Patients using doctors with hospital staff positions should be prepared to frequently start over with a new physician at times. In addition, the staff doctor is given guidelines by the hospital or clinic administration to see more patients more quickly—often within six to ten minutes per patient. This is not enough time for either the doctor or the patient to ask important questions and listen carefully to the answers.

Now that you know the basics of the bureaucracies that will make the rules and provide your care, you can be a more informed patient who understands how to find the best care.

How Best to Deal with Bureaucracies

- As frustrating as the experience of dealing with bureaucracies might be, remain empathetic when dealing with the people who work in these institutions. Many—I would say most—of them truly want to help people but are overworked and forced to see too many patients in too little time.

- Remember that you are building a team of caregivers. Aside from your family and friends, who we have discussed, your team should include the doctors, the employees in their offices, and the staff and administrators in the clinics, hospitals, and insurance companies.

- Have your paperwork ready. Everyone should have a written will, but as a patient, you need a health-care proxy that gives decision-making power about your care to someone you trust. In addition, your insurance information should always be with you.

- Learn from people who share your condition by contacting clinics or charities with that focus. Many will have patient support groups or counselors who will help you individually, generally at no cost. Find others who have coped with your illness and ask about their experiences managing the system. Learn from their successes and frustrations.

Five Guidelines for Choosing a Hospital

1. **You want to be in a hospital that treats many people with your condition.** Hospitals specialize in many areas, such as prostate cancer or heart problems. You want to be treated by a medical team that is familiar with your condition and expert in treating it.

2. **You want a hospital that has a strong reputation for providing excellent patient service.** We have all heard stories about patients who were left for hours waiting for their sheets to be changed or to have their IV line reconnected. You don't want that to be you. Find a high-service institution with a good nurses-to-patient ratio.

3. **You want the hospital where your doctor works.** If you carefully selected a doctor whose expertise, values, and people skills guided your choice, then you want to be either an outpatient in the clinic or an inpatient in the hospital with which your doctor is affiliated. Your doctor can then be your best advocate for excellent care from other staff members.

4. **Location, location, location.** While cell-phone and video calls are wonderful ways to stay in touch with the outside world, when you are hospitalized, nothing is as meaningful as a personal visit. At least that is how I feel. If you agree, choosing a hospital that is convenient for your friends and relatives may be important.

5. **Find the right vibe.** I really can't quantify "vibe" in specific terms, but in my experience as a patient and a visitor, some hospitals have a healing vibe. They are filled with sick people but sick people who seem to be getting better. Other hospitals may seem as if they are filled with suffering patients who are only getting worse. Given the choice, I want to be in a place with a healing vibe. I guess we can call this another type of chemistry test.

Chapter 13

CONFRONT YOUR DISEASE BY BEING MORE THAN A PATIENT

I have met people who revel in their disease. They treat it as some sort of badge of honor, almost boasting about the seriousness of their condition and the near torture they have endured to combat it. I feel like asking them if this disease and its treatment is what defines them. I just walk away from them feeling sorry that they don't see themselves as more than just a patient who finds little about themselves to celebrate other than their scary diagnosis and all that they subsequently endured.

Compare this person to some of the people you have met in this book, such as Don or Adam. There are some truly famous cases of people who received very scary diagnoses and yet went on to be inspiring optimists. Franklin D. Roosevelt contracted polio at the age of thirty-nine and would never walk again without the help of braces and crutches. But not being able to walk didn't stop Roosevelt from becoming governor of New York and president of the United States. Leading the country out of the Great Depression and guiding the Allies during World War II, he is credited by many historians as being one of America's greatest presidents. During his twelve years as president, Roosevelt became synonymous with optimism. When he spoke to the nation at the beginning of the war and said, "We have nothing to fear but fear itself," he might as well have been speaking about his own scary diagnosis.

The physicist Stephen Hawking was diagnosed with a form of ALS, or Lou Gehrig's disease, when he was twenty-one years old. He was told to expect not to live more than two years. Hawking died fifty-five years later. Throughout Hawking's life, ALS destroyed his ability to work, write, and feed himself. Within a few years he was wheelchair bound. Toward the end of his life, his only means of communication was through a computer that translated the movement of a single muscle in his cheek into letters and words. Yet his productivity remained extraordinary. Hawking developed groundbreaking theories of the universe, wrote bestselling books, and campaigned for greater accommodations for people with disabilities.

Ethan Skinner

Nearly 1.5 million Americans have type 1 diabetes (T1D) and over one hundred thousand people die from it each year, largely because it goes undiagnosed (Barbara Davis Center for Diabetes at the University of Colorado). Type 1 diabetes is an autoimmune disease in which a person's body destroys the cells in the pancreas that manufacture insulin. Without insulin, the body cannot process sugar for energy. As a backup, the body breaks down fat into ketones. High levels of ketones are life-threatening and account for a large number of the deaths from T1D.

Early symptoms include unquenchable thirst, mood changes, weight loss, dry skin, and pain from nerve damage.

Having type 1 diabetes or having a likelihood of developing it, is easily tested, but almost no one does so because most people don't see it as a distinct disease from type 2 diabetes, which tends to develop gradually in overweight adults with poor diets. Parents who don't know the difference between type 1 and type 2 often see a diagnosis of diabetes as a stigma and will fall into denial when a doctor tells them their child has diabetes.

People with type 1 are typically treated with insulin through self-administered injections into fatty tissue just below the skin, through pumps that monitor glucose levels in the blood and automatically inject insulin, or through inhalers. Proper treatment requires attentive and active management by patients because they may be testing their glucose levels several times during the day through finger-stick tests or glucose monitors held on the skin. Even some smartwatches can measure glucose levels. Because insulin is needed to process carbohydrates, patients need to monitor their carbohydrate consumption and use insulin accordingly. In addition, because blood sugar levels can fall with changes in eating or activity, patients need to watch for low blood sugar levels and eat to raise them as needed. Diabetes patients need to be their own first-line doctors, and having diabetes can take over a patient's life.

Ethan Skinner was always a parent's dream. He excelled at school academically and socially. He received top grades, had good friends, and was even voted the class clown by his classmates. But the bathroom next to his bedroom had a squeaky door. That squeaky door is actually central to Ethan's diagnosis.

When Ethan was thirteen, his mother, Teresa, noticed that Ethan was getting up to use the bathroom a number of times during the night. Perhaps this would be understandable if he were seventy, but not at thirteen. That planted a seed in her mind. Then a few weeks later, Ethan was changing shirts and Teresa was shocked at how skinny he was. She called the doctor's office and made an appointment for the upcoming Monday. He had lost fifteen pounds in the last year; and at five feet seven, he weighed under a hundred pounds. The doctor gave him a urine test and then told Ethan and his mom to go directly to the emergency room. Teresa, in shock, asked for a second opinion. The doctor said in a stronger voice, "Get to the emergency room."

The emergency room was the gateway to Ethan's new world as a type I diabetes patient. In fact, one of the doctors there opined that given the very high levels of ketones in Ethan's blood—a condition known as diabetic ketoacidosis (DKA)—if left untreated, Ethan could have died in a week. In the emergency room, Ethan was given insulin, which brought his blood sugar levels down to normal and removed him from danger. Ethan had just entered the world of a patient with a complex chronic disease. Fortunately for him, he was in one of the best places in the world to learn how to manage diabetes.

For many years, I was fortunate to receive my hemophilia care at a comprehensive care center at Mount Sinai Hospital in New York City. The concept of a comprehensive care center for any disease is that one doctor in one specialty is not sufficient to care for all the needs of patients with chronic illnesses. In addition to hematologists, the Comprehensive Hemophilia Treatment Center had orthopedists, internists, dentists, social workers, and nurses—all of whom were experienced in the care of hemophilia patients and who collaborated as a team.

The Barbara Davis Center for Diabetes at the University of Colorado near Ethan's home followed the same philosophy.

It provided education and treatment and carried out advanced research to improve diagnosis and treatment. One of their missions is to expand routine antibody testing of all children to identify type 1 diabetes and treat it before it becomes life-threatening. Type 1 diabetes can be identified with a simple blood test for autoantibodies.

As any parent of a teenager knows, exacting compliance from a teenager is a challenge. Whether it is about doing homework, staying away from drugs and alcohol, or picking up their rooms, it can be a struggle. For those with type 1 diabetes, compliance can be a matter of life and death.

Ethan accepted the guidance he received at the Barbara Davis Center and set himself on a course of helping others. But today at age twenty, he openly admits he had periods when he resented all the demands that diabetes made on him and his compliance would fall off. An A1C test is a measure of average glucose levels over a three-month period. After an A1C test showed Ethan had done a poor job of managing his glucose levels, his doctor told him that if he didn't improve the management of his diabetes, he could lose his sight or even a limb. After that discussion, Ethan became a model patient.

Ethan was well-equipped to be a model patient. He excelled in math and science in school, which helped him keep track of all the required testing and insulin adjustments. He was given an insulin pump, which delivers frequent microdoses of insulin as needed. He also wears a continuous glucose monitor (CGM), which measures glucose levels through a small needle put under his skin and changed every few days. The CGM talks to an app on his smartphone and with the insulin pump via Bluetooth so the pump can adjust its administration of insulin. Sounds seamless and automated. But it isn't.

These devices—as brilliant and advanced as they are—are not perfect and can't be blindly relied upon. Patients need to learn how they feel when their blood sugar goes too high or too low. In such cases, they have to go to manual backup, testing with finger sticks and injecting supplemental insulin, or eating something sweet to bring their glucose levels back in line. This also means carrying with them an array of tools: alcohol swabs, syringes, vials of insulin, finger-stick tools to extract a drop of blood, and inhalers that deliver insulin quickly if needed.

Sure, Ethan is a model patient, managing his diabetes flawlessly. But this is not Ethan's greatest accomplishment. Ethan has moved past his disease to lead a full and productive life. He was inspired by the caregivers at the Barbara Davis Center and decided to pursue a career in which he could help others. Today he is an emergency medical technician (EMT), answering calls for people in dire need, occasionally including patients with diabetes who didn't manage or couldn't obtain their insulin and were now in danger of dying from diabetic ketoacidosis (DKA).

Ethan also volunteers with the Barbara Davis Center to promote expanded testing for T1D, maintains his strong friendships, and has a girlfriend his mother thinks is wonderful. He has reached the point where he can now experience gratitude for how his diabetes has taught him to better understand his body. It has also led him to his profession as an EMT and his very satisfying volunteer work with the Barbara Davis Center.

No one would think a squeaky bathroom door would be the first step toward a life of gratitude and meaning, but for Ethan Skinner it was.

The list of people who overcame disabilities to lead full and productive lives is too long for this book. I will just mention a few familiar individuals: the legendary musicians Ray Charles and Stevie Wonder, and the author and educator Helen Keller. Like them, you have to accommodate but not collapse under the weight of your diagnosis. You can have chemotherapy treatments on Thursday and still enjoy a wonderful dinner with friends over the weekend. Having this attitude requires a strong dose of optimism.

Optimism is a bias that predisposes one to assume positive outcomes. This attitude, along with its inverse, pessimism, have long been studied and shown to have a significant impact on health, especially cardiovascular health such as heart disease and strokes. Some researchers believe that pessimism itself is exacerbated by stress, resulting in high blood pressure, insomnia, and a host of other conditions.

Everything about cancer and its treatment is big: big risks and major anxiety for the patient, large research studies for potential new drugs and diagnostic tests, big data from studies about the efficacy of new drugs, and—of course—huge costs at every step. Some of the most respected medical institutions in the world include Memorial Sloan Kettering in New York City, Dana-Farber Cancer Institute in Boston, the Cleveland Clinic, Mayo Clinic in Minnesota, and MD Anderson Cancer Center in Houston. For patients without access to such institutions, their only options may be hospitals and clinics with less experienced staff, limited access to the newest drugs, and providing care with older and less effective diagnostic equipment. As with every disease, having the best insurance and access to the best care greatly improves the odds of obtaining the best outcome.

Without insurance that pays $2,000 for monthly MRIs, or thousands of dollars monthly for the latest drug, or $25,000 for stem cell transplants, patients are pressed between suboptimal care or bankruptcy. Yet when a patient with excellent insurance finds a great doctor and hospital, the outcomes can be spectacular. The American Cancer Society reports that childhood leukemia, which once had a 90 percent fatality rate, now has a 90 percent cure rate. Myeloma ten-year survival rates have gone from less than 10 percent to over 30 percent in the last thirty years.

Michael Hamilton is a successful executive coach. He never had any significant health problems, and he had been an All-American tennis player who played competitively until his cancer diagnosis. Michael met his internist while playing tennis. The doctor impressed Michael at their first consultation, taking forty-five minutes rather than the typical ten for the office visit. He became Michael's family doctor for the next fifteen years. Michael referred to him as his Marcus Welby.

After Michael's forty-five-minute checkup, the doctor said that although Michael's tests were normal, he suspected the presence of a simmering health issue, and he suggested Michael return in three months. Without leaving room for discussion, Michael's wife said it was time for a second opinion from Memorial Sloan Kettering. Within a week, Michael was a patient there.

Myeloma is a cancer of the platelet blood cells, which are essential for proper clotting. These cells also play an important role in supporting the body's immune system. When the newly formed platelets are cancerous, they will not work properly, and they will produce proteins that damage the kidneys and create bone lesions. Untreated, myeloma will spread and is fatal. Sitting at the crossroads of chemotherapy and stem cell treatments, myeloma has received billions in research funding, which has produced significant improvements in patient outcomes.

Cancer patients face tasks as daunting as training for a triathlon. They need to manage a matrix of medications, side effects, lab tests, nutrition, and appointments with at least several specialists. Many cancer patients compromise on treatments to save money; others with advanced disease may choose palliative care over trying to cure their cancer.

Yet there are others who have the personal and financial resources to take on the challenge to defeat their disease without compromise and give themselves additional healthy years of life. Michael Hamilton chose to battle his cancer but without the expectation that he could cure it. His approach to managing his cancer was, as he puts it, "to kick the can down the road." He was just looking for more time. In this sense, he was a perfect match for the physicians at Memorial Sloan Kettering who told him that every round of treatment would buy more time, eventually enabling him to try effective new treatments in the future.

Michael started a triple-drug combination therapy that pushed his disease into remission without any significant side effects. He stayed on this therapy for three years. He also prepared for what might be the next level of treatment—a stem cell transplant. Stem cells are the foundational cells that seed the creation of blood and other cells. When myeloma advances, the next line of attack is to "restart" the immune system by first destroying the bone marrow where the cancerous blood cells are created and then reintroducing healthy stem cells back into the bone marrow. Before Michael's disease had advanced, his doctors harvested his healthy stem cells and froze them for this potential future use.

Three years after his initial diagnosis, tests showed that Michael's cancer had come back more forcefully and the doctors recommended a stem cell transplant. This first step requires drugs to destroy the unhealthy bone marrow, which left Michael without an immune system until his previously harvested stem cells could be transfused back into him. Throughout this process, Michael continued on chemotherapy. The procedure went well, and Michael recovered, but three months later, he developed a fever, became delirious, and was diagnosed with multiple bacterial and viral infections, a condition known as sepsis. His wife and daughter began to plan his funeral.

He began to recover again and was moved to a subacute care center where the nurses wore plastic bags because the COVID-19 pandemic had created shortages of proper medical garb. This facility's task was to help Michael regain his strength and be able to walk again.

He regained his strength, but other complications followed. He developed a gallstone, requiring minor surgery. On one of his visits to Memorial Sloan Kettering, he contracted COVID-19. Then a heart arrhythmia emerged but receded with some adjustments to his meds.

Today, Michael is back at home, working on various professional projects, grilling in the backyard, and puppy-sitting for his daughter's dog when she and her husband are out of town. He has had a few swings in his platelet count that have been dealt with through more adjustments to his chemo. Sometimes, he confesses, he becomes depressed, but that is rare. His wife is a superb and attentive manager; and Michael, perhaps from years of athletic training, is good at being coached. Michael says he is able to compartmentalize his medical issues from his family and professional lives, but this would not be possible without the partnership—and leadership—that his wife provides. Grateful as he is for her help, he also feels guilty that his health often requires her to put her needs on hold while she takes care of him.

Neither Michael nor his wife, Caren, expected years focused on health issues, but together they have managed Michael's health and their lives to maintain a current steady and happy state.

Always remember that you are in charge.

As you come to terms with your scary diagnosis, your thinking will vacillate between "It couldn't be worse" and "It could be worse."

I've been there. Until I was about twenty years old, my thoughts were focused on the "It couldn't be worse" side. I was focused on the activities I wanted to participate in but that my parents prohibited out of caution because of my hemophilia and serious injuries. As I became older, I missed those activities less and came to appreciate the intellectual and people skills that I possessed. This self-awareness made me more secure and confident. This shift was crucial. My thinking moved to the "It could be worse" side. Many of the people I have interviewed for this book shared similar stories with me.

As I have emphasized, one of the toughest parts of receiving a scary diagnosis is the loss of control—loss of control of your body, your treatment, your life. All of these are true to varying degrees until you finally realize that you are the ultimate and best decision-maker. Even in the face of a progressive disease, you can and should make the decisions about what treatments to undergo, how to manage your time and relationships, and how to focus on activities that take you away from your disease and connect to the real world.

Think of Don, who when he was diagnosed with Parkinson's disease decided to move back to his hometown of St. Louis because most of his family was there. He was not looking for caregivers. Rather, it was where the people he wanted to spend his time with were located. Think of Adam, the severely ill veteran who prayed for his own death while doubting he would ever recover. Adam found fulfillment in his life by helping other injured veterans find their paths to recovery. Or Deborah and Tom, the parents who had suffered one miscarriage, one baby who died shortly after birth, and the premature birth of their baby girl Abigail, who died after six months in intensive care. Without diminishing their losses, they refocused on building their family with the birth of a premature but healthy baby boy who now has a daughter of his own, a little girl he adores. Today, Deborah, after the death of her husband, is a doting grandmother.

These and other stories of perseverance have made me believe that given the choice between optimism and pessimism, most people naturally gravitate to optimism, gratitude, and hope.

There is a powerful duality about a scary diagnosis. It can bring the likelihood of negative outcomes, such as the inevitable progression of your disease or death. But it can also be an early warning of a condition that can be cured or successfully managed indefinitely.

Regardless of the prognosis, as you accept that you are not powerless and realize that it could have been worse, you have laid the foundation for feeling gratitude and optimism for the rest of your life. For many people, this confidence is fed by the availability of effective treatments. Medical advances have moved diseases such as HIV, many types of cancers, and kidney failure from being acute and quickly fatal to being chronic and manageable. Certainly this is something to be grateful for.

Everyone's life is finite, but a scary diagnosis brings mortality into clear focus. Whether we are dealing with an aggressive cancer for which there is no treatment or planning a long retirement with the knowledge that no member of our family in the last three generations has lived less than a hundred years, we must make the most of the time we have.

If this book leaves you with one enduring lesson following your scary diagnosis, I hope that you successfully move your thinking from "It couldn't be worse" to "It can be worse" and your attitude from pessimism to optimism. When you achieve that, a scary diagnosis will no longer be seen as tolling the end of your life. Rather, it will be a new journey that teaches you to become an expert manager, a person who asks the right questions, and someone who can accurately evaluate your doctor's skills—which will then enable you to make the best decisions.

When you can do that, you will receive the gifts of gratitude and optimism.

Chapter 14

WITH GRATITUDE, OPTIMISM IS SUSTAINABLE

I have seen several interviews with the actor Michael J. Fox, who now at the age of sixty-two has lived more than half his life with Parkinson's disease. Parkinson's is progressive and day by day it has taken away more of the charmed life Fox had as a young, successful star. Yet he has not lost touch with gratitude for all the good things about his life. As he put it in a May 1, 2023 interview on *CBS Sunday Morning*, "With gratitude, optimism is sustainable."

Fox speaks from the long and close relationship with his disease. Although I don't know him, I would expect that he arrived at this wise lesson over a period of years. Certainly that is what I have experienced following the scary diagnoses I have received.

In my twenties, I began to appreciate the community of people with hemophilia to which I belonged. I could see in others the courage and determination to prevent hemophilia from defining them and dominating their lives. Eventually I realized that I had some of those qualities, too. I also experienced the broader world in which I would no longer be judged by how well I played sports or roughhoused with my friends. I did well academically and was grateful that I was smart enough to excel in activities that were unimpeded by hemophilia, such as playing the cello or being on the bridge team. While the doctors who saw me as a young child judged my life expectancy to be less than twenty years, I have now beaten those estimates by more than fifty years. How can I not be grateful? But this process for me took a long time. If you have only recently received your scary diagnosis, you need a strategy to find *and* nurture your gratitude.

Your diagnosis has given you the opportunity to learn about yourself and to witness your strength and courage in the face of your diagnosis. For many, a scary diagnosis becomes an opportunity to connect with their religion and faith, appreciate the inspiring people with similar conditions that they have met, regrow connections to many friends and family that may have weakened over the years, and learn that there are many ways to find satisfaction at work, including working from home.

I previously introduced you to Adam Greathouse, an army veteran who was gravely injured in Kosovo, but let me share the details of his story. Adam's story is one of gratitude. For Adam Greathouse, his scary diagnosis thrust him into a state of fear and despair.

Adam was raised in rural West Virginia where opportunities were scarce. He graduated from high school and obtained a job at a small local factory. Being able to support his two children was the first taste of self-esteem Adam had ever experienced. After two years, the factory downsized and Adam's position was eliminated, so he and his children moved in with his parents.

His brief taste of self-esteem and accomplishment evaporated. At the age of twenty, he felt he was a failure.

Adam saw an army recruiting ad and thought that this might be the way back to supporting his children. He visited a recruiting office and learned that they would train him in fiber optic technology. He signed up and was sent to Fort Jackson in South Carolina for basic training, and then to Fort Stewart in Georgia to become skilled in the operation and maintenance of infantry communication equipment. In 2001, he was assigned to the NATO peacekeeping mission in war-torn Kosovo for a six-month tour of duty. His parents took over the care of his two children.

Adam believed that being a soldier was the high point of his life. He loved being part of a team, appreciated the rigid discipline of the military, and felt appreciated by his superior officers and the soldiers he supported by installing and maintaining their essential communication equipment. While out on patrol with British and Swedish observers, his convoy entered an area of active fighting. They escaped any direct fire by speeding back to the base as quickly as possible, kicking up clouds of dust from the dirt road they traveled.

Back in the barracks, Adam's commanding officer praised him for keeping the convoy communication equipment working during the episode. Adam began to feel weak and ill, but he joined some members of his unit for dinner. After eating, he walked weakly to his army cot and immediately fell asleep. Those would be the last unassisted steps Adam would take for five months. A medic in his unit recognized that Adam's disturbed sleep and gasping for air signaled a serious medical problem, so he arranged to rush Adam to the medical unit, where they gave him supplemental oxygen. But Adam didn't stabilize. His heart stopped and was restarted by CPR, during which Adam heard the doctor say that he couldn't stabilize him. Recognizing that Adam needed a higher level of medical care, the army mobilized a move to a facility with a higher level of care. This would save Adam's life.

The doctors never learned with certainty what caused Adam to become ill. Throughout the fighting in Kosovo, poison gas, similar to mustard gas, was used. The most effective treatment for exposure to mustard gas, which was used by Germany in World War I, was to quickly hose down soldiers with water. To accomplish this, the Allies created a fleet of tanker trucks that were brought to the front lines. If mustard gas stays on the skin or reaches other membranes, including lungs and eyes, it causes large and painful blisters within twenty-four hours of exposure. Since Adam was not hosed down immediately following his exposure, his symptoms took between twenty-four and forty-eight hours to appear. Because the hosing did not happen, doctors could only provide life-support while his body worked to clear itself of the poison.

Adam remembers being carried onto a C-130 transport plane but little else about the journey to the Landsthul Hospital, a medical center in Germany for US and coalition forces, Department of State personnel, and repatriated US citizens. Adam would spend the next months intubated and in a medically induced coma. During these first weeks at Landsthul, the doctors determined that large parts of Adam's lungs were too damaged to heal, so they operated, leaving him with about two-thirds of one lung. Adam also had an allergic reaction to the blood-thinner heparin, which is often given to patients after surgery to prevent dangerous blood clots. In Adam's case, the heparin caused his blood to clot uncontrollably, which is precisely the opposite of its intended effect. When he awoke two months later, he was numb from the waist down, and he saw that his once strong body had withered from a muscular 215 pounds to a frail 115 pounds. The doctors told him that the lack of oxygen in his body had likely injured his brain in ways that might only become apparent over time.

Adam overheard the staff making arrangements to send his dead body back to the States. There was already a chief petty officer from Fort Stewart assigned to accompany the body. The young man who joined the army to build a career, support his children, and find self-esteem now prayed for a quick death.

But Adam didn't die in that hospital in Germany, and he doesn't remember the flight home. His next memory was waking up in Walter Reed National Military Medical Center in Washington, DC, with his mother standing at the foot of the bed. It was there that he began the agonizingly slow work to rebuild his strength and eventually recover enough strength to go to his parents' home. Throughout his stay at Walter Reed, Adam's father stayed with him twenty-four hours a day, providing care and company. Although his body continued to slowly improve, Adam's mood worsened. He couldn't imagine being a productive person again and believed that he began this journey as a failure and ended it as a failure.

To numb his physical and mental pain, Adam turned to the original anesthesia—alcohol. He started drinking a fifth of whiskey every day. When he was able to drive again, he pointed his car at a big tree in hopes of ending his pain, but he didn't kill himself. Today he is thankful for failing at his attempted suicide.

Adam didn't hit the tree, but his failed suicide marked the beginning of a turnaround. He realized that he needed to find a more positive way to think about his situation. He stopped drinking, became more serious about his physical therapy, and began to see some reasons for optimism. Adam treated his recovery as a military mission in which soldiers are taught to "adapt and overcome." With the help and support of his family and the care team at the veterans hospital in West Virginia, he was able to acknowledge his gratitude for his family, his army training, and the help he was receiving.

Adam joined the recreational therapy programs sponsored by the Disabled American Veterans organization. They took him whitewater rafting and taught him how to snowboard and surf. In the process Adam became a person eager to embrace life. The social worker at the VA recognized that Adam was a thoughtful and articulate person and asked him to speak to other injured veterans. Today Adam is active in veteran organizations and travels to conferences and meetings throughout the United States.

Adam speaks eloquently about how he found gratitude, which connected him to his optimism, which in turn changed his life. He realizes that helping others find their gratitude and optimism is satisfying and important work, and Adam no longer thinks of himself as a failure.

As the gratitude your scary diagnosis has given you grows, your ability to look to the future with optimism also increases. Gratitude resides everywhere, even in the depths of fear, despair, and pain.

My fullest statement of my own gratitude I wrote to the family of the man whose liver I now carry. The organ donor system goes to great lengths to maintain the anonymity of organ donors and organ recipients. But it manages a system of writing to each other and then, if both agree, arrange an in-person meeting of the donor family and the recipient. Here is the letter I wrote to the donor's family. The donor's mother responded with a kind and touching note but declined to meet.

Dear Friends,

My wife has written to you and given you some of our background as it relates to coping with loss and also some of the background on my health history. I don't want to repeat that, but I do want to tell you about how profoundly I am affected—physically and emotionally—by the gift I have received. First of all, I physically feel great. Even though I didn't have clear outward signs of liver disease, I now think that perhaps more subtle signs had crept up on me slowly over the years and were hard to notice. Now with a healthy liver, I feel the difference. I am aware of this every moment and grateful for this gift of health.

On the emotional side, I am actually more affected. I have been given extraordinary gifts in my life—loving parents, two children who are beautiful inside and out, and an extraordinary and loving wife who I miss whenever I am not with her. I have a job I love and many wonderful friends. But no one has ever given me the gift of being able to continue this life—until my transplant.

I cannot imagine the grief that gripped you at the time of your loss. Yet you moved past this to think about others and to turn a terrible loss into something that had some positives. Nothing will, I am sure, ever make up for that loss. But your handling of this loss and your gift to me and others will always inspire me, move me, and change the way I live. Whenever I am confronted by a tough decision, I will think of your decision and how you rose to make something good come of it. In that way, the values and love of your family will continue with me.

I am grateful for your gift and the positive influences it has had and will always have on me. You gave me a liver and a continued life. But you also shared with me your way of living and loving. I am grateful for both.

Should you ever desire to meet me, it would be my pleasure to do so.

Dear Reader:

To those of you who have read this book, I also add my gratitude. Thinking of you and the issues you have been facing has motivated me through the process of writing. I sincerely hope that sharing my experiences and providing guidance has been useful and valuable to you.

Suggested Reading

Ledley, Fred D., Sarah Shonka McCoy, Gregoary Vaughn, Ekaterina Galkina Cleary. "Profitability of Large Pharmaceutical Companies Compared With Other Large Public Companies," JAMA, March 3, 2020.

Magee, Mike. *Code Blue: Inside America's Medical Industrial Complex*. New York: Grove Atlantic, 2019

Makary, Marty. *The Price We Pay: What Broke American Health Care—and How to Fix It*. New York: Bloomsbury, 2021.

_____. *Unaccountable: What Hospitals Won't Tell You and How Transparency Can Revolutionize Health Care*. New York: Bloomsbury, 2013.

Rosenthal, Elisabeth. *An American Sickness: How Healthcare Became Big Business and How You Can Take It Back*. New York: Penguin, 2018.

Index

A
ADA (Americans with Disabilities Act of 1990), 47
Aetna, 107, 109
Affordable Care Act of 2014 (Obamacare), 108–9, 111–12
agency. *See* personal agency
ALS, 124
alternative medicine, 18–19, 87
amateur physicians, 69
Americans with Disabilities Act of 1990 (ADA), 47
Anatomy of an Illness as Perceived by the Patient (book by Norman Cousins), 88
Anatomy of an Illness as Perceived by the Patient (film), 88
attitude. *See* mental attitude
attribution bias, 67–68
avoidance. *See* denial and depression

B
bad decisions. *See* flawed thinking
Barbara Davis Center for Diabetes, 126–27, 128
Barron, Ava, 35–37
biases, 26, 65–70, 129–30
Biden, Jill, 37
Biden, Joe, 37
bleeding disorders, 43–46. *See also* hemophilia
boundary setting, 96

C
cancer
    health insurance and outcomes, 129–31

kidney cancer, 35–37
leukemia, 15, 130
life expectancy, 15
myeloma, 129–32
pancreatic cancer, 18–19, 20
Candid Camera (TV show), 88
cardiovascular disease, 15–16
cause-and-effect thinking, 26–27
chemical poisoning, 9, 137–41
"chemistry" test, 73, 77–78, 83, 122
childhood leukemia, 130
children. *See* pediatric care
clear thinking guidelines, 70–71
Cleveland Clinic, 14, 98
COBRA insurance coverage, 107–8, 109
cognitive dissonance, 68
confirmation bias, 26, 67, 68
control. *See* agency
Cousins, Norman, 88
COVID-19, 132
Creutzfeldt-Jakob disease, 78–79

D

decisions
    biases and, 26, 65–70
    flawed thinking, 26–29
    guidelines for, 7, 70–71
    research and, 22, 26–27, 28
denial and depression
    about, 18–21, 29
    author's personal story, 22–26
    distrust and, 69 (*See also* distrust and suspicion)
    medication side effects, 22–24
    risky behavior and, 25–26
    strategies for addressing, 21–22
diabetes, 124–28
diabetic ketoacidosis (DKA), 126
diagnosis. *See* scary diagnosis
diagnostic errors, 11–12
dignity
    author's personal story, 57–64

tools for maintaining, 57–58, 64
disabilities, 47–48, 92–93, 123–28, 129–30
Disabled American Veterans organization, 141
distribution companies, 119
distrust and suspicion
   biases, 65–70
   guidelines for, 70–71
doctors
   author's personal story, 2–4, 74–82, 84–85
   bureaucracy and, 119–20, 122
   "chemistry" test for, 73, 77–78, 83
   choosing a doctor, 73–74, 77–78, 82–83
   communication skills, 78–82, 84–85
   distrust and suspicion of, 65–71
   guidelines for visit preparations, 31–32
   personal agency and, 72–73
   preconceptions, 30–32
   rankings of, 5–6
   self-interests of, 5–6, 74, 83
   specialists, 82
   training of, 82–83
Dokken, Deborah, 39–41, 134

E
Education for All Handicapped Children Act of 1975 (EAHCA), 47–48
Ephron, Nora, 93

F
faith and hope, 84–91. *See also* gratitude; mental attitude
   author's personal story, 61–62, 84–87
   gratitude and, 137
   laughter as medicine, 85, 88, 91
   positive attitude, 16, 29–33, 87–88, 91, 96
   religious experiences, 61–62, 86–87, 90–91, 137
   resilience, 85–86, 89–90
   sources of, 91
   team members and, 88–89, 91
family-and-friends team
   author's personal story, 50–52
   decision making by, 27

faith in, 88–89, 91
gratitude for, 140–41
guidelines for, 21, 22, 64, 71, 101
hospital visits from, 101
medical leave laws, 95–96
members of, 54–56
parents caring for children, 36–37, 40–42, 46–47, 48 (*See also* pediatric care)
perseverance stories involving, 132–34
sharing health information with, 95
spouses, 52–54, 132–33

fear
author's personal story, 13–14, 61
denial and, 20–22, 25
distrust and, 67, 68, 69, 70
optimism vs. fear, 124, 137–41
parental, 39, 51
prayer for, 61
therapy for, 55

Federal Family and Medical Leave Act (FMLA), 95–96
flawed thinking, 26–29
Fox, Michael J., 136
friends. *See* family-and-friends team

G

generic drugs, 118–19
Gibbel, Mark, 107–8
gratitude, 136–43
   author's personal story, 136–37, 141–43
   military veterans' story of, 137–41
   optimism as sustainable with, 136, 141
Greathouse, Adam, 8–9, 14–15, 134, 137–41

H

Hamilton, Michael, 130–33
Hawking, Stephen, 124
health-care system bureaucracy, 106–22
   background, 6–7, 106–7
   distribution companies, 119
   distrust and suspicion of, 65–71
   doctors, 119–20, 122 (*See also* doctors)

guidelines for dealing with, 120–21
hospitals, 116–17, 121–22 (*See also* hospital experience)
nonprofit organizations, 111
preconceptions of, 29–33
private companies, 110–11, 114, 117–19
public organizations, 111–12, 114, 115–16
single-payer insurance, 114
health insurance
business model, 5, 112–13, 115
cancer outcomes and, 129–31
changing types of, 107–9
employment-related, 107, 109, 115
organization types, 111–12, 114–15
self-interests of insurance companies, 5, 11–12
single-payer insurance, 109–10, 114
heart disease, 15–16
hemophilia, 2–4, 13–14, 42–46, 58–63, 74–76, 92–94, 136–37
hepatitis C, 22–24, 74–75
hope. *See* faith and hope
hospital experience, 97–105
author's personal story, 13–14
bureaucracy and, 116–17, 121–22
comprehensive care centers, 126–27
customer service, 99–100
guidelines for choosing, 121–22
guidelines for maintaining sanity, 100–101
rankings of, 6, 97–98
roommates and their guests, 101–5
self-interests of hospitals, 6, 98–100
types of, 14–15, 98, 140
humor, 85, 88, 91

I
Individuals with Disabilities Education Act (IDEA), 47–48
inner circle. *See* family-and-friends team
insurance companies. *See* health insurance
interferon, 22–24
Isaacson, Walter, 20
"It could be worse," 133–35

J
Jobs, Steve, 18–19, 20

K
Kahneman, Daniel, 65–66
kidney cancer, 35–37
kidney stones, 108, 109
Kim-Schluger, Leona, 76, 80, 84, 85

L
laughter as medicine, 85, 88, 91
Leopold (prince), 44
leukemia, 15, 130
life expectancy, 15–16, 19–20, 86
liver diseases and transplant, 2, 7, 13–14, 22–24, 76–81, 84–85, 141–43
losing dignity. *See* dignity
Lou Gehrig's disease, 124
lymphoblastic leukemia, 15

M
mad cow disease, 78–79
made-up symptoms, 69–70
Medicaid, 109, 111–12, 114
medical errors, 11–12, 38
medical leave laws, 95–96
Medicare, 109, 111–12, 114, 118
medications, 22–24, 117–19
Memorial Sloan Kettering, 35–37, 130, 131–32
mental attitude. *See also* faith and hope; fear; gratitude; pessimism; positivity
   life expectancy statistics, 15–16
   process following diagnosis, 13–15
   for taking action, 16–17, 29–33, 87–88, 91, 96, 129, 136, 141
   (*See also* personal agency)
military veterans, 8–9, 14–15, 115–16, 134, 137–41
Mount Sinai Hospital, 13–14, 75–77, 80, 126
Munchausen Syndrome, 69–70
mustard gas, 139
myeloma, 130–31

N

New School for Social Research, 107–8
New York Hospital, 76
Nicholas II (tsar), 45
nonprofit organizations, 111

O

Obamacare (Affordable Care Act), 108–9, 111–12
optimism, 16–17, 87–88, 91, 96, 129, 136, 141. *See also* faith and hope; gratitude; mental attitude
organ transplant. *See* liver diseases and transplant

P

pancreatic cancer, 18–19, 20
paranoia. *See* distrust and suspicion
Parkinson's disease, 10, 52–54, 90–91, 134, 136
pediatric care, 34–49
   author's personal story, 42–47, 48, 57–64
   background, 34–35, 46
   guidelines for, 49
   hospitals dedicated to, 38–39
   kidney cancer diagnosis, 35–37
   leukemia diagnosis, 15, 130
   parental actions, 36–37, 40–42, 46–47, 48
   premature babies, 39–40
   rehabilitation and education, 47–48, 92–93
personal agency
   author's personal story, 6–7, 133
   background, 1–3, 7
   cancer outcomes and, 129–33
   doctors and, 72–73
   health insurance coverage and, 129–31
   "It could be worse," 133–35
   optimism and, 16–17, 129
   overcoming disabilities, 123–28
personal chemistry test, 73, 77–78, 83, 122
personal resilience, 63, 64, 85–86, 89–90
pessimism, 13, 56, 129, 134–35
pharmaceutical companies, 110–11, 117–19

pharmaceutical distribution companies, 119
pharmacies, 119
physicians. *See* doctors; hospital experience
polio, 123–24
positivity, 16, 29–33, 87–88, 91, 96, 129, 136, 141. *See also* faith and hope; gratitude; mental attitude
post-traumatic stress disorder, 63, 64
preconceptions
   denial and depression, 18–26, 29, 69
   flawed thinking, 26–29
   guidelines for challenging, 27–28
   hope, 29–33 (*See also* faith and hope)
   of medical system, 29–33
prejudice, 66–67, 68–69
privacy, 92–96, 101–5
processing diagnoses
   first steps, 10–11, 12
   second opinions, 3, 11–12
   uncertainty and, 8–11
public hospitals, 116
public organizations, 111–12

Q
questioning behavior. *See* distrust and suspicion

R
Rasputin, Grigori, 45
Reagan, Ronald, 108
recreational therapy programs, 141
Rehabilitation Act (1973), 47
rehabilitation and education, 47–48, 92–93, 123–28
religious experiences, 61–62, 86–87, 90–91, 137. *See also* faith and hope
research
   for decision making, 22, 26–27, 28
   drug development, 117–18
resilience, 63, 64, 85–86, 89–90
respect. *See* dignity
risky behavior, 25–26
Romanov, Alexei Nikolaevich, 45
Roosevelt, Franklin D., 47, 123–24

S

scary diagnosis
  for children. *See* pediatric care
  health-care system and, 4–6 (*See also* doctors; health-care system bureaucracy; hospital experience)
  losing dignity, 57–64
  processing diagnoses, 3, 4, 8–12
  responses to, 1–2, 7, 13–17 (*See also* dignity; distrust and suspicion; faith and hope; gratitude; mental attitude; personal agency; preconceptions)
  second opinions for, 3, 11–12, 71
  sharing, 92–96
Schepers, Don, 52–54, 86, 90–91, 134
second opinions, 3, 11–12, 71
self-inflicted symptoms, 69–70
sharing scary diagnoses, 92–96
single-payer insurance, 109–10
skepticism, 28
Skinner, Ethan, 124–28
Social Security, 111–12
stem cell transplant, 131–32
Steve Jobs (Isaacson), 20
suicidal thoughts, 22–24, 140–41

T

team members. *See* doctors; family-and-friends team
thinking errors, 26–29
Thinking Fast and Slow (Kahneman), 66
The Three Stooges Show, 85, 88, 91
Truman, Harry, 114
type 1 diabetes (T1D), 124–28

U

UnitedHealthcare, 107, 108, 109
U.S. military hospitals, 14–15

V

Veterans Administration health-care system, 111–12, 115–16, 141. *See also* military veterans
Victoria (queen), 44–45

von Willebrand disease, 43–44
vulnerability. *See* preconceptions

W
Walsh, Christopher, 75–76, 80
Washington, George, 11
workplace, 95–96